NUTRI-TIPS

NUTRI-TIPS

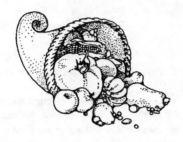

BRIAN MORGAN, Ph.D.

AND

ROBERTA MORGAN

LONGMEADOW PRESS

Cover design by Lisa Amoroso

Interior design by Fritz Metsch

Morgan, Brian L. G.
    Nutri-tips / Brian Morgan and Roberta Morgan.
        p.   cm.
    ISBN 0–681–41184–8
    1. Food—Composition.   2. Nutrition.   I. Morgan,
Roberta, 1953–.
    II. Title.
TX531.M65   1992
641.5′63—dc20   91–27931
                                                          CIP

ISBN: 0–681–41184–8

Printed in the United States of America

First Edition

0 9 8 7 6 5 4 3 2 1

ACKNOWLEDGMENTS

We would like to thank Samuel Mitnick of The Mitnick Agency, and Pam Altschul of Longmeadow Press.

DEDICATION

To Brian, from Roberta
To Roberta, from Brian

Our best friend, love, support and
inspiration is each other.

CONTENTS

Preface: How to Use this Book

The purpose of this book is simple—to make selecting the right foods for you and your family as effortless as possible. Let's say you're preparing a salad for the following guests:

> Harry, who has a heart condition, and has to eat foods low in fat and cholesterol;
>
> Rita, his wife, who is 30 pounds overweight and on a strict weight-loss diet;
>
> Susan, Rita's sister, with a blood pressure problem that necessitates a low salt diet;
>
> and Jeffrey, Susan's boyfriend, who has just found out he's anemic and has been advised to eat foods high in iron.

What would you put in that salad?

While most guests don't pose this many problems at once, many families are now eating cholesterol, calorie, or salt-restricted diets just to maintain better health. You can prepare that salad (which might contain spinach leaves, fresh green and yellow vegetables, apples, apricots, and lemon juice dressing) with ease and with considerable flair by using this book. Just look up the salad foods that come to mind and you will easily see whether they're low in fat, salt, calories, etc., and high in nutrients like iron or vitamin C. In addition, good and bad points about these foods are included—things you wouldn't ordinarily think about—like the fact that artichokes can cause skin rashes in certain susceptible, allergic people. This would warn you to ask about certain foods while serving new guests, or planning the perfect lunch at your favorite restaurant!

You can also flip through the entries to get some ideas about which foods to choose for your friends' and family's particular nutrient needs . . . or just which foods to choose for optimal health benefits.

1

SERVING SIZES

The serving sizes will vary from food to food. Wherever it is possible, we have chosen measures for each food that can be easily spotted (such as one medium-sized apple). The nutritional values for each food are then calculated according to the serving size—in other words, if we say that apples contain 120 mg of potassium, we are saying that one medium-sized apple contains 120 mg. Naturally, a larger apple will have more.

THE USRDA

The amount of a nutrient that any food contains is listed according to its percentage of the USRDA (except where there is no RDA value for the food). Although we may use the term RDA, we are actually referring to the values of the USRDA. The difference is that the RDA, or Recommended Daily Allowance, may have a few values for a specific nutrient, whereas the USRDA always takes the highest value. For example, men require 11 mg of iron and women 18, according to the RDA. The USRDA is the highest amount, or 18 for both men and women. We have chosen this system so you can be sure that everyone in the family is getting enough of the nutrient.

THE NUTRIENTS

We have not listed every nutrient contained in a food, but only the ones that exist in a large enough quantity to make a difference to your diet. There may be traces of other vitamins or minerals which are not mentioned in the entry because the amount contained is insignificant and has no real health impact, either for good or bad.

THE RATING SYSTEM

You will notice that each food has been listed with a "star rating"—from no stars to four—which should give you an initial impression of how good the food is for your health. The system is calculated as follows:

NO STARS—This is a food that has little or no nutritional value but may have major drawbacks, such as being high in fat and calories. If you can, stay away from these foods.

★ONE STAR—This is a food with some nutritional value, but with major drawbacks, such as being high in sodium or saturated fat. Eat these foods only in moderation, and if you are on a special diet—such as one that restricts fat, sodium or caloric intake—you will probably want to avoid most of them.

★★TWO STARS—These either have good nutritional value, but some important drawbacks, as well; or few drawbacks, but not great value. They can usually be safely enjoyed by everyone, but check the "bad points" section to make sure there is not something about them that would restrict their use in your particular case (such as a food that causes an allergic reaction you may susceptible to, or one that has a few too many calories).

★★★THREE STARS—These are the beneficial foods, with few drawbacks and high nutritional value. Eat as many of them as you can on a daily basis. The only bad points they may have are either minor or specific to only certain people (such as rare allergic reactions).

★★★★FOUR STARS—These foods boost your health in a variety of ways and, apart from rare allergic reactions, don't really have any drawbacks. The more of these you can work into your diet, the better you'll feel, look, breathe, etc.

Of course, no diet would be very interesting, or balanced for that matter, if you ate only "four-star" foods. However, there is usually no reason to select a one-star food or one without any benefits at all. Try to stick to those with over two stars as much as you can. There is no doubt about the fact that what you eat can affect every facet of your life—how you feel, think, work, sleep, and look—so to be at your best, eat the best.

AN ADDITION TO YOUR KITCHEN, OR YOUR BRIEFCASE

While no one wants to brag, we will dare to say that anyone who cares about their health, who wants to diet, who needs to eat certain foods and avoid others, will find this book an indispensable guide. It summarizes a wealth of nutrition and dietary information in the simplest and most useful format. We hope you will feel the same.

Dr. Brian Morgan
Roberta Morgan
New York and Miami 1991

Nutrients and How They Work

What is the good of the food you eat? Each nutrient has its own role to play in the proper growth, development, maintenance and repair of the body. That is why a balanced diet is so important—to make sure all these crucial jobs are getting done on a daily basis. In the entries which follow, you will learn which foods are high in beneficial nutrients. Use the information below to see what these nutrients do for your health and appearance.

Vitamin A is needed for healthy eyes, bones, hair, glands, nails, and a strong immune system. Carotene is converted by the body into vitamin A; consuming it may lower your risk for getting cancers of the larynx, esophagus and lungs. The USRDA (Recommended Daily Allowance) for this vitamin is 1000 RE's (Retinol Equivalents—the most modern measure of vitamin A) or 5000 IU's.

The B Complex Vitamins

   B1, also called thiamine (USRDA = 1.5 mg), is needed to break down carbohydrate in the body, for muscle coordination and for healthy nerve tissue.

   B2 (USRDA = 1.7 mg), also called riboflavin, helps the body convert proteins, fats, and carbohydrates into energy, and is needed for growing tissues, keeping existing tissues healthy, and for maintaining the health of the skin and eyes. A lack of vitamin B2 in your diet, will make your eyes appear bloodshot.

   B3 (USRDA = 20 mg) also called niacin, helps to convert the food we eat into energy and makes fat, which is used in the replacement of worn-out cells.

   B6 (USRDA = 2 mg) also called pyridoxine, is

needed for the breakdown of dietary proteins, the formation of certain body proteins, and the proper functioning of the nervous system. Too little B6 in the diet can lead to depression and may be implicated in disorders like premenstrual syndrome.

B12 (USRDA = 6 mcg) is needed for the normal development of red blood cells and for the healthy functioning of all cells, particularly those in the bone marrow, nervous system, and intestines.

FOLIC ACID (USRDA = 400 mcg) is needed for the formation of nucleic acids—RNA and DNA, the genetic material found in all the cells of the body—as well as for the normal use of food proteins, the replacement of worn-out red blood cells and, like iron, the prevention of anemia. Too little folic acid in the diet can lead to bleeding gums.

PANTOTHENIC ACID (USRDA = 10 mg) plays a crucial role in our ability to get energy from the food we eat, and helps the body make fat, a necessary part of all our cells. Deficiencies in this B vitamin make a person more susceptible to infection, impair the ability to sleep, and cause general aches and pains, the sensation of "pins and needles," and numbness in the hands.

Vitamin C (USRDA = 60 mg) is important for healthy teeth, gums, blood vessels, bones and as protection against disease. It also aids in iron absorption, and may help protect your body against cancer. While some of the other claims about this vitamin— that it cures the common cold, for instance—have not been proven, it is still essential to your health. Women who take oral contraceptives, smokers, and people with chronic gum disease may be deficient in vitamin C.

Calcium (USRDA = 1000 mg) is needed to build bones and teeth and to keep bones strong; 99% of the body's calcium is found in these structures. The bones also form a reservoir of calcium used to maintain blood calcium at a constant level. The remainder helps to keep cell membranes healthy, helps transport substances in and out of cells, helps pass messages to and from muscles and around the nervous system, and is essential for normal blood clotting and the activation of many enzymes. Calcium also helps to keep your blood pressure in the normal range. Women have to be especially careful to take in enough every day (or run the risk of developing osteoporosis, or brittle bones, after menopause).

Carbohydrates come in two forms: simple and complex. A simple "carb," like the refined sugar in your coffee, contains just calories that the brain uses for fuel. However, simple sugars can cause tooth decay. Complex carbohydrates, found in foods like pasta, potatoes, cereals, bread, squash, and nuts are rich in other nutrients (such as the B vitamins) and are also an essential energy source. In fact, as much as 50–60% of your dietary calories should come from complex carbohydrates.

Copper (USRDA = 2 mg) is involved in the absorption and use of iron by the body. A copper deficiency can lead to anemia. It is also a part of many enzymes in the body that help extract energy from the food we eat.

Vitamin D (USRDA = 400 IU's) has as its major function regulating calcium and phosphate use by the body, which is needed for the development of healthy and strong teeth and bones. You get most of your daily requirement for this vitamin from the sun. The USRDA is 400 IU's.

Vitamin E (USRDA = 30 IU's or 10 mg) helps protect our cell membranes from wear and tear, and may help heal wounds when applied topically. It may also prevent the formation of "free radicals" in the body, chemical substances that could be involved in causing cancer.

Fiber helps our digestion and prevents many gastrointestinal disorders, such as constipation and diverticulosis. It also reduces your risk for developing cancer of the large intestine. One form of fiber called PECTIN can lower blood cholesterol levels by reducing the absorption of fat. Pectin is also good for people with diarrhea, because it helps to solidify the stools. While there is no RDA for fiber, you should ideally take in 10 to 15 grams a day.

Iodine (USRDA-150 mcg.) is needed by the thyroid gland to enable it to produce thyroid hormone, which controls the rate that the cells in the body work, as well as the general growth and development of children.

Iron (USRDA-18 mg.) is an integral part of hemoglobin in the blood and myoglobin in the muscles, which supply the cells with oxygen. It is also a part of many enzymes and proteins in the body. If you take in too little iron, you could end up with a sallow complexion, brittle nails, falling hair, fatigue, and anemia.

Vitamin K is needed for the manufacture of certain substances in the liver responsible for blood clotting. Deficiencies in this vitamin are rare. While there is no RDA value, you need from 70 to 140 mcg daily.

Magnesium (USRDA-400 mg.) is essential for bone growth, the manufacture of body proteins, the liberation of energy from carbohydrates, and the workings of the nerves and muscles.

Phosphorus (USRDA-1000 mg.) helps build strong bones and teeth. It is important for the release of energy from carbohydrates, proteins, and fats, and assists in the formation of new cells and enzymes.

Potassium is a natural diuretic and works against the water-retaining properties of sodium. It is also important for the nervous system, the muscles, and helps in the body's conversion of food into energy. There is no RDA for potassium, but you should ideally take in from 4 to 5 grams a day.

Protein (USRDA-45–65) grams is essential to the building of new cells, the repair of worn-out tissues, and the manufacture of neurotransmitters, enzymes, and hormones. It is also important for healthy skin and muscles.

Zinc (USRDA-15 mg.) is involved in the manufacture of new cells and body proteins. It assists in the proper action of the hormone insulin (which affects blood glucose levels), and is essential for the normal functioning of the immune system. It also is required for the sense of taste.

THE CULPRITS IN
YOUR DIET

Just as there are good things in the food you eat, there are also substances on your plate that can do minor or serious damage to your health. It may not be enough to eat healthy items when you are still eating unhealthy ones. For example, a person with high cholesterol can actually be shortening his life by consuming a lot of fatty meat and eggs, even if he is also taking in omega-3 fatty acids and pectin, which tend to lower blood cholesterol levels. However, even the culprits in your diet often have their purpose, provided they are not eaten to excess. Below are the nutrients with "mixed attributes":

CALORIES
Calories are units of energy. Too many of them in your diet can lead to a weight problem, which in turn can result in serious illnesses such as diabetes. An average woman needs about 1500 calories per day and an average man needs 2500. These figures vary depending on the size of the person and their level of activity.

CHOLESTEROL
Cholesterol is a building block of all cell membranes. It also plays essential roles in the manufacture of bile (which helps you absorb fat), of sex hormones (estrogen, progesterone, and testosterone), of vitamin D, and of myelin (the fatty sheath that insulates the nerves). However, cholesterol is produced in the liver and intestines at a rate sufficient to meet the body's needs. In most people, the more cholesterol consumed, the less the body makes, a system that works very well as long as you take in 150 to 300 mg daily. Eating more than this may lead to an increase in blood cholesterol levels. If blood cholesterol rises above 180 mg per 100 ml of blood serum (in other words, a total cholesterol reading of 180) your risk of

having a stroke or heart attack is increased (2% for every 1% rise in cholesterol).

FAT

Fats are composed of substances called fatty acids. Saturated fats are generally hard in consistency at room temperature; monounsaturated fats are soft at room temperature and harder when refrigerated; polyunsaturates are liquid at room and refrigerator temperatures. Saturated fat elevates blood cholesterol levels, while the other two types tend to lower it. However, consuming any type of fat seems to raise your risk of getting cancer, especially cancers of the colon, breast, ovary, endometrium, cervix, and prostate. Your body only requires 1 to 2% of your daily caloric intake as a particular kind of polyunsaturated fat (found mainly in vegetable oils) called linoleic acid, which forms a part of all cell membranes in the body. The amount of fat you take in can therefore safely be reduced to no more than 30 percent or less of your total caloric intake, with equal parts being monounsaturated, polyunsaturated, and saturated.

SIMPLE CARBOHYDRATES (SUGARS)

Simple carbohydrates are a source of empty calories, providing energy but very little else in the way of essential nutrients. Although it has been said that sugars cause a number of health problems—such as hyperactivity in children and hypoglycemia in adults—their only proven health hazard is that they can cause tooth decay if consumed in quantity without brushing one's teeth shortly afterwards.

SODIUM

Sodium is required for the normal functioning of the nerves and muscles and in the transport of essential nutrients across cell membranes. From our knowledge of its function in the body, it appears that an adult needs about 1/2 gram (500 mg) of sodium daily, or less than 1/4 of a teaspoon of salt a day. Ideally, no one should consume more than 3 grams (3000 mg) daily. An increased consumption of salt (sodium chloride) increases the absorption of salt into the blood, which attracts fluid into the bloodstream and increases the amount of circulating fluid in the blood vessels. This causes an increased demand on the kidneys to excrete both the excess salt and fluid. Should the kidneys fail to do this, the heart must work harder to pump all the added fluid. This may eventually lead to the development of hypertension (high blood pressure) and its complications, such as heart disease and strokes. Roughly one in five Americans are sensitive to the blood pressure elevating effects of sodium. Excess consumption of salt can also cause edema (swelling of the tissues).

Sodium is one of the mineral nutrients found in almost all the plants and animals we consume as food. The average level of consumption in the U.S. diet is estimated at 6 to 8 grams per day—approximately two to three times higher than it should be. That amount is equivalent to three to four tablespoons of table salt. People who do not usually add salt to their food may still be taking in more sodium than they imagine: commercially-processed foods have 1.6 to 2.3 grams; plant and animal foods naturally contain 1 to 2 grams; even drinking water contains 0.05 to 0.25 grams per quart. You should avoid adding salt to food, and check labels on food products to see how much sodium they contain. Those on seriously restricted salt diets have to watch what they eat even more carefully.

THE COMPLETE A-Z GUIDE TO FOOD

ALMOND

Serving Size: 1 ounce
Rating: ★★

CALORIES: 170
FAT: 16 grams
B COMPLEX VITAMINS: 18% for B2, 7% for folic acid
CALCIUM: 8%
VITAMIN E: 60%
FIBER: 4 grams
IRON: 7%
MAGNESIUM: 20%
PHOSPHORUS: 13%
POTASSIUM: 258 mg
PROTEIN: 8%
ZINC: 6%

GOOD POINTS
Almonds are especially good for their nutritional value. They are very high in fiber, potassium, and vitamin E (which might make them potent "anti-cancer" foods). They also contain significant amounts of vegetable protein, calcium, phosphorus, magnesium, iron, zinc, folic acid and vitamin B2. A sprinkling of almonds on top of a salad, main course, or dessert is a healthy and tasty accent.

BAD POINTS:
Almonds are high in fat and calories. (Dieters definitely should not munch on handfuls of al-

monds!) Since the fat is in the form of monounsaturated and polyunsaturated fat it tends to lower your blood cholesterol levels, but any fat seems to raise your risk of breast, uterine, endometrial, ovarian, prostate, and colon cancer.

APPLE

(WITH SKIN)

Serving Size: 1 medium
Rating: ★★

CALORIES: 80
FAT: 0.5 grams
SIMPLE CARBOHYDRATES: 20 grams
VITAMIN C: 12% (most is found right under the skin).
FIBER: 9–10 grams; about 25% of it is in the form of pectin, which can lower blood cholesterol levels by reducing the absorption of fat.
POTASSIUM: 160 mg

GOOD POINTS

Apples are low in fat, which means that they can be eaten with safety by people with heart disease. They are also low in sodium, which makes them an ideal fruit for low salt diets because of high blood pressure or water retention (as in sufferers of PMS). However, when buying dried apples beware of those treated with sodium sulfur compounds: they are very high in sodium.

This fruit is also low in calories, high in potassium and fiber, and contains significant amounts of vitamin C (especially good for those who need to boost their C intake, such as women on birth control pills, smokers, and people with chronic gum disease). Apples make great sweeteners for meals and salads and are perfect after-dinner snacks for both dieters and people eating "heart smart" foods.

BAD POINTS

Raw apples can cause FLATULENCE (gas), because the indigestible fiber may be broken down by bacteria in the large intestine. Bruised apples contain a potentially dangerous substance called PATULIN, which, if consumed in very large quantities over many years, may cause liver cancer. Dried apples are sometimes sprayed with SULFITES to preserve them. Some people are allergic to sulfites, and could develop symptoms such as rashes, watery eyes, and breathing problems.

Apple seeds contain AMYGDALIN, a naturally-occurring substance that breaks down into hydrogen cyanide. While accidentally swallowing the occasional seed is not a problem, taking in a large number of seeds could be hazardous and even a few seeds could be lethal in a very small child. Apples also contain some simple carbohydrate, which can promote tooth decay.

Apricots

*Serving Size: Three medium (fresh)
or six halves (dried)
Rating: ★★*

CALORIES: 40
SIMPLE CARBOHYDRATES: 9.5 grams
VITAMIN A (AS CAROTENE): 20%
POTASSIUM: 365 mg
FAT: 0.4 grams

GOOD POINTS

Apricots are low in fat, which means that they can be eaten with safety by people with heart disease. Fresh and dried apricots are also low in sodium, which makes them an ideal fruit for people on low salt diets. However, when buying dried apricots beware of those treated with sodium sulfur compounds because they are very high in sodium.

Apricots are low in calories, and contain significant amounts of vitamin A (in the form of carotene, possibly an "anti-cancer" food) and potassium. They can give an extra special taste to any meal, and can be nibbled happily by dieters and health-conscious eaters.

BAD·POINTS

Apricot pits contain AMYGDALIN which breaks down into hydrogen cyanide in the stomach and could be fatal if consumed in large quantities. Dried apricots are sometimes sprayed with SULFITES to preserve them. Some people are allergic to these substances and could develop symptoms such as rashes, watery eyes and breathing problems. Apricots also contain some simple carbohydrate, which can promote tooth decay.

ARTICHOKE

Serving Size: 1 large
Rating: ★★

CALORIES: 44
FAT: 0.1 grams
VITAMIN C: 13%
CALCIUM: 4–5%
COMPLEX CARBOHYDRATE: 8 grams
FIBER: 2–3 grams
IRON: 6%
POTASSIUM: 300 mg

GOOD POINTS

Artichokes are low in fat, calories, contain no cholesterol and contain a lot of vitamin C, potassium, calcium, iron, and fiber. They make a nice appetizer, side dish, or can be added to meals and salads.

BAD POINTS

Artichokes contain CYNARIN, a sweet-tasting substance that dissolves in the saliva and can sweeten the taste of everything you eat right afterwards. They also contain oils that can cause a skin rash in susceptible people, known as CONTACT DERMATITIS. If the artichokes are not fresh but packaged in oil, they can be higher in fat and calories.

ASPARAGUS

Serving Size: ²/₃ cup (pieces, cooked)
Rating: ★★★

CALORIES: 20
FAT: 0.3 grams
VITAMIN A (AS CAROTENE): 18%
B COMPLEX VITAMINS: 11% for B1, 11% for B2, and 7% for B3
VITAMIN C: 43%
VITAMIN E: 25%
POTASSIUM: 180 mg

GOOD POINTS

This vegetable is a good source of vitamins A, B1, B2, B3, C, E, and potassium. It is low in calories, contains no fat, and is one of the foods that many experts feel may reduce your risk of getting cancer.

BAD POINTS

Canned, rather than fresh boiled or steamed asparagus can be very high in SODIUM (370 mg) and should be avoided by people on salt restriction diets. When you eat asparagus your body excretes into the urine a compound called METHYL MERCAPTAN, which has an unpleasant odor.

AVOCADO

Serving Size: 1 medium
Rating: ★

CALORIES: 306
FAT: 30 grams
VITAMIN A (AS CAROTENE): 21%
B COMPLEX VITAMINS: 13% for B1, 12% for B2, 17% for B3, 25% for B6, 28% for folic acid, and 17% for pantothenic acid.
VITAMIN C: 25%
COPPER: 25%
VITAMIN E: 33%

FIBER: 3.7 grams
IRON: 11%
MAGNESIUM: 18%
POTASSIUM: 1097 mg
ZINC: 5%

GOOD POINTS
Avocados are a rich source of potassium, copper, and vitamins A, E, and C. They contain significant amounts of fiber, magnesium, zinc, iron, and B complex vitamins. Since B6 is a nutrient recommended by many doctors to women with premenstrual problems, avocados filled with shrimp or chicken salad may be an idea lunch for PMS sufferers. They are also delicious on salads—as long as you aren't on a strict diet.

BAD POINTS
Avocados are very high in fat (it comprises 22% of their weight), although over 80% of it is in the form of monounsaturated and polyunsaturated fat, which lowers blood cholesterol and helps reduce the risk of heart disease. However, the consumption of large amounts of any type of fat appears to increase the risk of getting certain types of cancers, including ovarian, endometrial, breast, prostate, and colon cancer.

By virtue of their high fat content, avocados are also high in calories. This is certainly a food to be avoided if you are on a diet.

Since they contain quite a bit of a substance called TYRAMINE, anyone taking the category of drugs known as monoamine oxidase inhibitors (MAOI's) should not eat them. This interaction can cause blood pressure to climb to a dangerous level.

BACON
Serving Size: 1 slice (crispy)
Rating: Sorry, no stars

CALORIES: 35
CHOLESTEROL: 5 mg
FAT: 3 grams
SODIUM: 114 mg

GOOD POINTS
None.

BAD POINTS
Bacon, when cooked to its full crispy glory, adds absolutely nothing good in the way of nutrients to your diet. However, it does contain some calories, salt, cholesterol and fat (mostly saturated) all of which can increase your risk of getting cardiovascular disease.

BAGEL

Serving Size: 1 whole
Rating: ★★

CALORIES: 163

FAT: 1.4 grams

SODIUM: 198 mg

B COMPLEX VITAMINS: 14% for B1, 9% for B2, and 10% for B3

COMPLEX CARBOHYDRATE: 31 grams

IRON: 8%

PROTEIN: 14%

GOOD POINTS
Bagels are not without nutritional value, containing significant amounts of the B complex vitamins, protein, and iron. They are tasty wrapped around just about any filling, from the traditional lox and cream cheese to cold chicken cutlets with lettuce and tomato.

BAD POINTS
Bagels contain a lot of calories and so would not be included on any slimming diets. They are also pretty high in sodium and so should be eaten in moderation by anyone on a salt-restricted diet.

BAKED BEANS

Serving Size: 3.5 ounces (canned in tomato sauce
Rating: ★★

CALORIES: 64

FAT: 0.5 grams

COMPLEX CARBOHYDRATE: 5 grams

SIMPLE CARBOHYDRATE: 5 grams

SODIUM: 480 grams

B COMPLEX VITAMINS: 6% for B6, and 7% for folic acid

COPPER: 10%

FIBER: 7.3 grams; some of it is in the form of pectin, which reduces blood cholesterol

IRON: 8%

POTASSIUM: 300 mg

PROTEIN: 8%

GOOD POINTS

Baked beans are an excellent source of fiber, for the prevention of constipation and other related gastrointestinal disorders. They also contain significant amounts of protein, copper, potassium, iron, vitamin B6 and folic acid, and are very low in calories. Since the fiber in them fills you up, they make a great diet food. Heap plenty on your plate to keep your mind and stomach away from higher calorie foods.

BAD POINTS

You only require 480 mg of sodium each day and one portion of baked beans just about does it!

The fiber in beans may cause FLATULENCE, since it is broken down by bacteria in the intestines. This food also contains some simple carbohydrate which can promote tooth decay.

BANANA

Serving Size: 1 medium
Rating: ★★★

CALORIES: 76
FAT: 0.4 grams
COMPLEX CARBOHYDRATE: 3 grams
SIMPLE CARBOHYDRATE: 16 grams
B COMPLEX VITAMINS: 26% for B6, 6% for folic acid
VITAMIN C: 17%
COPPER: 5 %
MAGNESIUM: 11%
POTASSIUM: 350 mg

GOOD POINTS
This tasty fruit is a good source of potassium, copper, magnesium, folic acid, and vitamins C and B6 (making them a smart food choice for those who may need a little more of the latter vitamin, such as PMS sufferers).

BAD POINTS
Bananas contain some simple carbohydrate, which can promote tooth decay.

BASS

(STRIPED, BROILED)

Serving Size: 3.5 ounces
Rating: ★★★

CALORIES: 228
FAT: 13 grams
B COMPLEX VITAMINS: 10% for B1, 8% for B2, and 15% for B3
IODINE: 10%
IRON: 11%
PROTEIN: 45%

GOOD POINTS
This is a highly nutritious food, containing good quality protein and significant amounts of the B

complex vitamins, iodine, and iron. For a main course, it is also not especially high in calories.

BAD POINTS
This fish contains significant quantities of fat, but of a kind known as omega-3 fatty acids, which tend to lower blood cholesterol levels. Fish is sometimes the cause of ALLERGIC SYMPTOMS such as stomach upset, hives, and swelling of the face, lips and eyes.

BEAN SPROUTS

Serving Size: 3.5 ounces (raw)
Rating: ★★

CALORIES: 35
FAT: none
B COMPLEX VITAMINS: 9% for B1, 8% for B2
VITAMIN C: 32%
COMPLEX CARBOHYDRATE: 7 grams
IRON: 1.3 mg
PHOSPHORUS: 6%
POTASSIUM: 220 mg
PROTEIN: 8%

GOOD POINTS
Bean sprouts are a very good source of vitamin C. They also contain significant amounts of B1, B2, (needed for energy and clear eyes), and are low in calories. Bean sprouts are a healthy addition to salads and a common component of Chinese dishes.

BAD POINTS
All raw beans and bean sprouts contain substances that inhibit the enzymes responsible for breaking down proteins and starches; substances that inactivate vitamin A; and substances called hemagglutinins that cause blood to clot. Happily, these substances are destroyed when the beans or bean sprouts are heated.

BEANS, GREEN
(FRENCH, STRING)

Serving Size: 1 cup raw
Rating: ★★★

CALORIES: 30

FAT: 0.3 grams

VITAMIN A: 14%

B COMPLEX VITAMINS: 6% for B1, 6% for B2, 6% for B3, 5% for B6, and 19% for folic acid

VITAMIN C: 25%

FIBER: 3.6 grams; some of it is in the form of pectin, which lowers blood cholesterol

IRON: 6%

MAGNESIUM: 9%

POTASSIUM: 350 mg

GOOD POINTS

Green beans are great "anti-cancer" foods, being rich in carotene, vitamin C, and fiber. Their high folic acid content can help prevent anemia and gum disease, and the fiber they contain prevents gastrointestinal problems and fills up the dieter. They are low in calories, and high in the B complex vitamins, iron, magnesium, and potassium.

BAD POINTS

The fiber in beans may cause FLATULENCE since it is broken down by bacteria in the intestines. All raw beans contain subbstances that inhibit the enzymes responsible for breaking down proteins and starches; substances that inactivate vitamin A; and substances called hemagglutinins that cause blood to clot. Happily, these substances are destroyed when the beans are heated.

BEANS, KIDNEY
Serving Size: ²/₅ cup (cooked)
Rating: ★★★

CALORIES: 118
FAT: .45 grams
B COMPLEX VITAMINS: 7% for B1, 25% for folic acid
COMPLEX CARBOHYDRATE: 21 grams
FIBER: 1.5 grams; some of it is in the form of pectin, which lowers blood cholesterol
IRON: 13%
PHOSPHORUS: 14%
POTASSIUM: 340 mg
PROTEIN: 12%

GOOD POINTS
Kidney beans contain a lot of protein, which makes them a wise food choice for the vegetarian. They are also a good source of B1, iron, phosphorus, potassium, fiber, and folic acid. (About one third of all young American women have less than optimal amounts of folic acid in their diets.)

BAD POINTS
The fiber may cause FLATULENCE, since it is broken down by bacteria in the intestines. All raw beans contain substances that inhibit the enzymes responsible for breaking down proteins and starches; substances that inactivate vitamin A; and substances called hemagglutinins that cause blood to clot. Happily, these substances are destroyed when the beans are heated.

Kidney beans contain a moderately high amount of calories.

BEANS, LIMA
Serving Size: ⁵/₈ cup (cooked)
Rating: ★★★

FAT: 0.3 grams
VITAMIN A: 6%
B COMPLEX VITAMINS: 12% for B1, 6% for B2, 7% for B3

VITAMIN C: 28%

COMPLEX CARBOHYDRATE: 20 grams

FIBER: 1.8 grams; some of it is in the form of pectin, which lowers blood cholesterol

IRON: 14%

PHOSPHORUS: 12%

POTASSIUM: 422 mg

PROTEIN: 12%

GOOD POINTS

Lima beans are a very good source of vitamin C, needed for healthy gums and possible protection against cancer. They also contain significant amounts of iron, fiber, the B complex vitamins, vitamin A, potassium, phosphorus, and are a good choice for vegetarians because they are high in protein.

BAD POINTS

The fiber may cause FLATULENCE, since it is broken down by bacteria in the intestines. All raw beans contain substances that inhibit the enzymes responsible for breaking down proteins and starches; substances that inactivate vitamin A; and substances called hemagglutinins that cause blood to clot. Happily, these substances are destroyed when the beans are heated. Lima beans also contain a moderately high amount of calories.

BEANS, SOY

Serving Size: ¹/₂ cup (cooked)
Rating: ★★★

CALORIES: 130

FAT: 6.3 grams

B COMPLEX VITAMINS: 14% for B1, 5% for B2, 28% for B3, and 29% for B6

CALCIUM: 7%

COMPLEX CARBOHYDRATE: 11 grams

FIBER: 1.6 grams; some of it is in the form of pectin, which lowers blood cholesterol levels

IRON: 15%

PHOSPHORUS: 18%

POTASSIUM: 540 mg
PROTEIN: 20%

GOOD POINTS
This food is the best source of vegetable protein in terms of quality and quantity—a must for all vegetarians. Soy beans also contain significant amounts of the B complex vitamins (especially B3 and B6) as well as healthy helpings of fiber, calcium, iron, phosphorus, and potassium.

BAD POINTS
The fiber may cause FLATULENCE, since it is broken down by bacteria in the intestines. All raw beans contain substances that inhibit the enzymes responsible for breaking down proteins and starches; substances that inactivate vitamin A; and substances called hemagglutinins that cause blood to clot. Happily, these substances are destroyed when the beans are heated.

Soy beans contain a moderately high amount of calories.

BEEF
(LEAN, COOKED)

Serving Size: 3.5 ounces
Rating: ★★★

CALORIES: 192
CHOLESTEROL: 82 mg
FAT: 9 grams
B COMPLEX VITAMINS: 5% for B1, 18% for B2, 30% for B3, 17% for B6, 33% for B12, and 10% for pantothenic acid
COPPER: 10%
IRON: 12%
MAGNESIUM: 6%
PHOSPHORUS: 19%
POTASSIUM: 350 mg
PROTEIN: 62%
ZINC: 37%

GOOD POINTS

Beef often gets a bad name. Although it does pose some problems, it's not a terrible food and is actually an excellent source of many nutrients. For a main course, it is also not especially high in calories. Beef provides us with the finest quality protein, is our best source of iron (vegetable iron is absorbed about one-third as well), and is a major source of vitamin B12 (found only in animal products). It also contains high amounts of the other B complex vitamins, phosphorus, zinc, copper, and potassium, as well as some magnesium. You should always make sure your beef is lean and trimmed of as much fat as possible, and people on cholesterol-restricted diets should not eat it more than once a week.

BAD POINTS

Beef contains a moderate amount of fat and a lot of cholesterol. A daily intake of more than 300 mg of cholesterol tends to raise the level in the blood and increase your risk of having a heart attack or stroke.

If you like to cook your beef out of doors, you should know that any barbecued food can contain CANCER-CAUSING AGENTS. The high temperatures char the fat and the resulting compound can contribute to the development of cancer. However, if you eat barbecued food infrequently, this is not a cause for concern.

BEER

Serving Size: 12 fluid ounces (1 glass)
Rating: Sorry, no stars

ALCOHOL: 13 grams

CALORIES: 148

FAT: none

SIMPLE CARBOHYDRATE: 14 grams

B COMPLEX VITAMINS: 9% for B3, 9% for B6, and 5% for folic acid

COPPER: 15%

IRON: 6%

MAGNESIUM: 9%

GOOD POINTS

Beer contains significant amounts of the B vitamins, magnesium, copper, potassium, phosphorus, and iron. (But if you think this sounds good, check out the bad points!)

BAD POINTS

The alcohol content depletes the body of vitamins A, B1, B2, B6, D, folic acid, calcium, magnesium, zinc, and glucose. It is also high in calories (although some beers, like light ones, will contain slightly less and dark ones may contain a little more). Beer contains some simple carbohydrate, which can promote tooth decay.

BEETS

Serving Size: 1/2 cup (cooked, diced)
Rating: ★

CALORIES: 25
FAT: none
VITAMIN C: 8%
POTASSIUM: 172 mg

GOOD POINTS

Beets contain some potassium, a small amount of vitamin C, and are low in calories. They make a tasty addition to salads, a nice basis for a cold summer soup, or a colorful side dish, but they are not quite as nutritious as many people think.

BAD POINTS

Beets contain NITRATES, which are converted in the body into NITRITES and NITROSAMINES— potential carcinogens (cancer-causing agents). If the beets are fresh, this is not a problem, but if they are cooked and left standing for some time at room temperature, bacteria that convert nitrates to nitrites multiply and the level of nitrites rises significantly.

BISCUIT

CALORIES: 93
FAT: 3 grams (but can be as high as 7 grams)
SODIUM: 262 mg
B COMPLEX VITAMINS: 8% for B1, 6% for B2
CALCIUM: 6%
COMPLEX CARBOHYDRATE: 14 grams
PHOSPHORUS: 13%
POTASSIUM: 56 mg

GOOD POINTS

Biscuits contains small amounts of vitamins B1 and B2, calcium, and potassium, along with a significant amount of phosphorus, but not enough of anything nutritious to justify their drawbacks as a snack or breakfast food.

BAD POINTS

Biscuits are high in sodium and so should be avoided by people with high blood pressure or a tendency to water retention. They also contain twice as much phosphorus as calcium which will prevent most of the calcium from being absorbed and used by the body. Biscuits are also high in calories, and saturated fat (which can raise your cholesterol levels). It also contains a substance called GLUTEN which can cause an upset digestive system, anemia, weight loss, back pain, skin problems, and water retention in people with a condition known as celiac disease.

BLACKBERRIES

Serving Size: 1/2 cup
Rating: ★ ★ ★

CALORIES: 37
FAT: 0.3 grams
SIMPLE CARBOHYDRATE: 9 grams
VITAMIN C: 25%

COPPER: 5%

FIBER: 3 grams; some of it is in the form of pectin, which lowers blood cholesterol

POTASSIUM: 141 mg

GOOD POINTS

This fruit is rich in vitamin C and low in calories, making it an excellent source of that vitamin when you are on a diet. In addition, blackberries contain a significant amount of fiber (which fills you up), potassium (a natural diuretic), and some copper (which helps prevent anemia).

BAD POINTS

Blackberries can case an **ALLERGIC REACTION** in susceptible people, resulting in symptoms like hives, stomach upset, and swelling of the face, lips, and eyes. They also contain some simple carbohydrate, which can promote tooth decay.

BLUE CHEESE

Serving Size: 1 ounce
Rating: ★★

CALORIES: 100

CHOLESTEROL: 21 mg

FAT: 8.2 grams

SODIUM: 396 mg

B COMPLEX VITAMINS: 6% for B2, 6% for B12

CALCIUM: 15%

PHOSPHORUS: 11%

POTASSIUM: 73 mg

PROTEIN: 14%

ZINC: 5%

GOOD POINTS

Dairy products are the best dietary source of calcium, needed for healthy bones and teeth among other things. They are also a good place to find some protein, which makes them important for both growing children and adults. Blue cheese also contains vitamin B12, phosphorus, potassium and zinc.

Being high in fat, calories, and cholesterol, this is not a good food choice for either dieters or people worried about their blood cholesterol levels. It is also high in sodium. People affected by LACTOSE IN-TOLERANCE lack an enzyme called lactase in their bodies, which is needed to break down milk sugar (lactose). As a result, when they eat dairy products, the lactose passes through the digestive system where it is broken down by bacteria instead, causing flatulence, bloating, and diarrhea.

BLUEBERRIES

Serving Size: 1/2 cup
Rating: ★★

CALORIES: 41
FAT: 0.3 grams
SIMPLE CARBOHYDRATE: 10 gram
VITAMIN C: 16%
FIBER: .95 mg; some of it is in the form of pectin, which lowers blood cholesterol
POTASSIUM: 65 mg

GOOD POINTS
Blueberries are a good source of vitamin C and are low in calories. They also contain some fiber and potassium.

BAD POINTS
Blueberries can cause an ALLERGIC REACTION in susceptible people, resulting in symptoms like hives, stomach upset, and swelling of the face, lips, and eyes. They also contain some simple carbohydrate, which can promote tooth decay.

BLUEFISH

Serving Size: 3 ounces (baked in margarine)
Rating: ★★★★

CALORIES: 135
FAT: 4 grams
B COMPLEX VITAMINS: 6% for B1, 5% for B2, and 8% for B3
IODINE: 10%
PHOSPHORUS: 24%
PROTEIN: 49%

GOOD POINTS
Bluefish is an excellent source of very good quality protein and at the same time is low in fat and calories. It also contains the B complex vitamins, iodine, and phosphorus. For heart-smart eaters, fish is one of the best foods you can select, and non-fatty fishes like bluefish are great for the waistline as well.

BAD POINTS
Fish is sometimes the cause of ALLERGIC SYMPTOMS such as stomach upset, hives, and swelling of the face, lips and eyes.

BOLOGNA
(BEEF)

Serving Size: 1 slice
Rating: Nope, no stars

CALORIES: 72
CHOLESTEROL: 13 mg
FAT: 6.5 grams
SODIUM: 230 mg
VITAMIN B12: 5%
PROTEIN: 6%

GOOD POINTS
You might choose chicken or fish filet sandwiches instead of the traditional version with bologna! It

might be tasty, but this lunch-time meat doesn't contain much—only a small amount of protein and vitamin B12.

BAD POINTS
Bologna is high in saturated fat and cholesterol—the wrong choice for cardiovascular fitness. It contains a lot of calories and sodium, which makes it wrong for slimmers and people on salt restricted diets, as well.

BRAN
(WHEAT)

Serving Size: 1 ounce
Rating: ★★★★

CALORIES: 104

FAT: 3 grams

B COMPLEX VITAMINS: 18% for B1, 6% for B2, 45% for B3, 20% for B6, 20% for folic acid, and 8% for pantothenic acid

COMPLEX CARBOHYDRATE: 12 grams

COPPER: 33%

FIBER: 13.2 grams

IRON: 22%

MAGNESIUM: 39%

PHOSPHORUS: 36%

POTASSIUM: 350 mg

PROTEIN: 7%

ZINC: 32%

GOOD POINTS
Bran is just a wonderful food choice, full of B complex vitamins, iron, and copper for energy, zinc for healthy skin, fiber for regularity, and magnesium and phosphorus for healthy bones. It also contains potassium and protein.

BAD POINTS
It contains a moderately high amount of calories, as well as a substance called GLUTEN which can cause an upset digestive system, anemia, weight loss, bone

pain, skin problems, and water retention in people with a condition known as celiac disease.

BRAZIL NUTS

Serving Size: 4 medium
Rating: ★★

CALORIES: 93
FAT: 9 grams
VITAMIN B1: 10%
VITAMIN E: 5%
FIBER: 1.4 grams
MAGNESIUM: 16%
PHOSPHORUS: 9%
POTASSIUM: 114 mg

GOOD POINTS
Brazil nuts are a good source of fiber (for a healthy digestive system), magnesium and phosphorus (for healthy bones), and vitamin B1 (for energy). They also contain good amounts of potassium and vitamin E. Mixed nuts make much more nutritious snacks than cakes, cookies, and candies, but if you're on a slimming diet, they're not much better.

BAD POINTS
Nuts are high in polyunsaturated fat. Nuts are also high in calories and, of course, salted nuts are very high in sodium. Brazil nuts can cause an ALLERGIC REACTION in susceptible people, resulting in symptoms like hives, stomach upset, and swelling of the face, lips, and eyes.

BREAD
(WHOLE WHEAT)

Serving Size: 1 slice
Rating: ★★

CALORIES: 61
FATS: 1 gram
SODIUM: 159 mg
COMPLEX CARBOHYDRATE: 11 grams
FIBER: 0.4 grams
IRON: 5%

GOOD POINTS
Bread is a good "fiber" food—it is a source of energy, in the form of starch, with very little fat. It also contains some vitamin B1, B3, and iron, and a moderate amount of calories. All commercially-made breads (white, whole wheat, rye, etc.) have about the same nutrient value except for one major difference: whole wheat has about twice as much fiber.

BAD POINTS
Most commercially-made breads are high in sodium. Also, bread contains several substances that could cause ALLERGIC REACTIONS or an upset digestive system, such as LACTOSE and GLUTEN.

BREWER'S YEAST

Serving Size: 1 tablespoon
Rating: ★★★★

CALORIES: 28
FAT: 0.05 grams (almost none)
B COMPLEX VITAMINS: 100% for B1, 25% for B2, 19% for B3
IRON: 9%
MAGNESIUM: 6%
PHOSPHORUS: 18%
POTASSIUM: 190 mg

GOOD POINTS

This food, usually in powder form, is an excellent source of the B complex vitamins, needed to supply the body with energy. It also contains significant amounts of iron, magnesium, phosphorus and potassium, and is relatively low in fat and calories. Mix it into food or cereal for a real health boost!

BAD POINTS

Yeast can cause FLATULENCE.

BROCCOLI

Serving Size: 1 large stalk (cooked)
Rating: ★★★★

CALORIES: 18
FAT: 0.3 grams
VITAMIN A: 25%
B COMPLEX VITAMINS: 12% for B2, 7% for B6, and 28% for folic acid
VITAMIN C: 57%
VITAMIN E: 9%
CALCIUM: 10%
FIBER: 3.6 grams
IRON: 8%
MAGNESIUM: 5%
PHOSPHORUS: 7%
POTASSIUM: 340 mg

GOOD POINTS

Broccoli is believed to reduce your risk of getting cancers of the respiratory tract and gastrointestinal system by virtue of its high carotene and vitamin C content, and by substances called DITHIOTHIONES that are found in all cruciferous vegetables (vegetables belonging to the cabbage family). Broccoli is also an excellent source of folic acid (which helps protect you against anemia and gum disease) and is low in calories. In addition, it contains generous amounts of calcium, magnesium, phosphorus, iron, potassium, fiber, and vitamins B2, B6, and E.

BAD POINTS

All cruciferous vegetables contain GOITROGENS—substances that hamper the production of thyroid hormones by the thyroid gland. This can cause an enlargement of the gland (goiter) in an attempt by the body to compensate for the reduced production by increasing the amount of tissue available. However, people with healthy thyroids would have to eat a very large amount of these vegetables before they would have any kind of problem. This is only of concern for those with sluggish thyroid glands. Goitrogens break down when the vegetable is heated, and so even if you have a thyroid problem, you can eat as much of the cooked vegetables as you want.

BRUSSELS SPROUTS

Serving Size: 6 to 8 medium (cooked)
Rating: ★★★

CALORIES: 18
FAT: 0.2 grams
VITAMIN A: 5%
B COMPLEX VITAMINS: 6% for B2, 9% for B6, and 22% for folic acid
VITAMIN C: 67%
FIBER: 2.9 grams
PHOSPHORUS: 5%
POTASSIUM: 240 mg

GOOD POINTS

Brussels sprouts are an excellent source of vitamin C and contain carotene, both of which are believed to give you some protection against GI and respiratory tract cancer. Cruciferous (belonging to the cabbage family) vegetables also contain dithiothiones, which offer additional protection. Brussels sprouts are low in calories, and a good source of folic acid, fiber, potassium, phosphorus, and vitamins B2, B6, and E. This is another excellent vegetable to eat on a regular basis.

BAD POINTS

All cruciferous vegetables contain GOITROGENS—substances that hamper the production of thyroid hormones by the thyroid gland. This can cause an enlargement of the gland (goiter) in an attempt by the body to compensate for the reduced hormone production by increasing the amount of tissue available. However, people with healthy thyroids would have to eat a very large amount of these vegetables before they would have any kind of problem. This is only of concern for those with sluggish thyroid glands. Goitrogens break down when the vegetable is heated, and so even if you have a thyroid problem, you can eat as much of the cooked vegetables as you want.

Brussels sprouts can cause FLATULENCE in some people.

BUTTER
(SALTED)

Serving Size: (1 tablespoon)
Rating: Sorry, no stars

CALORIES: 108
CHOLESTEROL: 33 mg
FAT: 12 grams
SODIUM: 123 mg
VITAMIN A: 9%

GOOD POINTS
What can we say about butter? Well, it's a good source of vitamin A.

BAD POINTS
What else can we say about butter? It is high in saturated fat and cholesterol. Salted butter also contains a lot of sodium as well as calories.

CABBAGE

Serving Size: 3/5 cup
Rating: ★★

CALORIES: 20
FAT: 0.2 grams
VITAMIN A: 5%
VITAMIN C: 55%
FIBER: 0.8 grams
FOLIC ACID: 12%
POTASSIUM: 163 mg

GOOD POINTS
Cabbage is an excellent source of vitamin C and contains carotene, both of which may protect you against respiratory and GI tract cancer. Being a cruciferous (belonging to the cabbage family) vegetable, it also contains dithiothiones, that offer additional protection. Cabbage has significant amounts of folic acid, potassium, and fiber, and is low in calories. A good vegetable choice.

BAD POINTS
All cruciferous vegetables contain GOITROGENS—substances that hamper the production of thyroid hormones by the thyroid gland. This can cause an enlargement of the gland (goiter) in an attempt by the body to compensate for the reduced hormone production by increasing the amount of tissue available. However, people with healthy thyroids would have to eat a very large amount of these vegetables before they would have any kind of problem. This is only of concern for those with sluggish thyroid glands. Goitrogens break down when the vegetable is heated, and so even if you have a thyroid problem, you can eat as much of the cooked vegetable as you want. Cabbage can cause FLATULENCE in susceptible people.

CAKE
(SPONGE)

Serving Size: 1 piece
Rating: ★

CALORIES: 181

CHOLESTEROL: 60 mg

FAT: 3.1 grams

COMPLEX CARBOHYDRATE: 13.6 grams

SIMPLE CARBOHYDRATE: 18.5 g

VITAMIN A: 5%

B COMPLEX VITAMINS: 5% for B1, 8% for B2

VITAMIN D: 6%

IRON: 6%

PHOSPHORUS: 9%

POTASSIUM: 72 mg

PROTEIN: 10%

GOOD POINTS
Cake contains a significant amount of protein and lesser amounts of vitamins A, B1, B2, and D, iron, phosphorus, and potassium. However, its drawbacks make this a poor way of getting these nutrients.

BAD POINTS
It should come as no news to anyone that cake is very high in calories. It is also high in simple carbohydrates (which can contribute to tooth decay), cholesterol, and contains GLUTEN, which can cause an allergic reaction in susceptible people. And, of course, toppings boost the caloric, fat, and cholesterol content even higher. The richer the cake is, the worse it is for your health.

CANDY
(HARD)

Serving Size: 3 pieces
Rating: Nope, no stars

CALORIES: 48
FAT: 0.1 grams
SIMPLE CARBOHYDRATE: 12 grams

GOOD POINTS
None, except perhaps that it is low in fat.

BAD POINTS
Candy is just a source of simple carbohydrate (sugar), which can cause tooth decay. And along with the sugar come lots of empty calories without any other nutrients to make them worthwhile.

CANDY BAR

Serving Size: 1 ounce bar
Rating: Nope, no stars

CALORIES: 129
FAT: 5 grams
SIMPLE CARBOHYDRATE: 18 grams
POTASSIUM: 67 mg

GOOD POINTS
Candy bars differ widely in content, but on the whole the only thing of value that most of them contribute to the body in significant quantities is potassium.

BAD POINTS
Candy bars are high in simple carbohydrate (which can cause tooth decay), contain significant amounts of unsaturated fat and saturated fat (which can contribute to the development of cardiovascular disease), and are high in calories.

CARAMEL

Serving Size: 3 pieces
Rating: No stars

CALORIES: 120
FAT: 5 grams
SIMPLE CARBOHYDRATE: 20 grams
SODIUM: 57 mg
POTASSIUM: 65 mg

GOOD POINTS

Caramels contain significant amounts of potassium, but because of their drawbacks, you'll probably want to get this nutrient from other foods.

BAD POINTS

These sweets contain a lot of simple carbohydrate and are especially bad for the teeth, because the caramel sticks there and can remain for long periods of time, providing an excellent breeding ground for the bacteria that cause tooth decay. They are also high in calories and contain significant amounts of fat and sodium.

CARROT

Serving Size: ²/₃ cup (cooked)
Rating: ★★★

CALORIES: 31
FAT: 0.1 grams
VITAMIN A (AS CAROTENE): 210%
FIBER: 1 gram, some of which is in the form of pectin, which lowers blood cholesterol
POTASSIUM: 222 mg

GOOD POINTS

These excellent snacking, salad, or side-dish vegetables are full of vitamin A (as carotene) which can give you some protection against cancers of the digestive and respiratory tract, as well as keeping your eyes, hair, and skin in top shape. They also contain a healthy amount of potassium and a little fiber, and are low in calories.

BAD POINTS
If you eat large amounts of carrots for extended periods your skin will take on a YELLOW APPEARANCE (as the fat in your body, including the fat under your skin, absorbs the yellow carotene).

CARROT JUICE
Serving Size: 1 cup (8 fluid ounces)
Rating: ★★

CALORIES: 96
FAT: 0.4 grams
SIMPLE CARBOHYDRATE: 21 grams
VITAMIN A: 230%

GOOD POINTS
Carrot juice is high in vitamin A (see CARROTS). Other than that, it really doesn't boast the nutritious value that some health-fad advocates like to believe.

BAD POINTS
Carrot juice is quite high in calories and has a lot of simple carbohydrate that can increase your risk of getting tooth decay. In addition, if you drink large amounts of carrot juice for extended periods your skin will take on a YELLOW APPEARANCE (as the fat in your body, including the fat under your skin, absorbs the yellow carotene).

CASHEWS

Serving Size: 6 to 8 (roasted)
Rating: ★

CALORIES: 84
FAT: 7 grams
MAGNESIUM: 10%
PHOSPHORUS: 6%
POTASSIUM: 70 mg

GOOD POINTS
Cashews contain significant amounts of potassium, phosphorus, and magnesium, but because of their high caloric content are not a good food choice for these nutrients.

BAD POINTS
They are high in fat and calories. Cashews can also cause an ALLERGIC REACTION in susceptible people, resulting in symptoms like hives, stomach upset, and swelling of the face, lips, and eyes.

(If the cashews are salted they will contain a lot of sodium.)

CAULIFLOWER

Serving Size: 1 cup (raw, pieces)
Rating: ★★★

CALORIES: 13
FAT: 0.1 grams
B COMPLEX VITAMINS: 7% for B1, 6% for B2, 10% for B6, and 10% for folic acid
VITAMIN C: 100%
FIBER: 2.1 grams
MAGNESIUM: 6%
POTASSIUM: 350 mg

GOOD POINTS
Cauliflower is an excellent source of vitamin C, and so is good for your gums and as protection against

cancer. Additional cancer protection comes from the dithiothiones it contains, found in all cruciferous (belonging to the cabbage family) vegetables. It is low in calories and has significant amounts of fiber, vitamins B1, B2, B6 and folic acid, magnesium and potassium.

BAD POINTS

The fiber is broken down by bacteria in the intestines and can cause FLATULENCE. All cruciferous (belonging to the cabbage family) vegetables contain GOITROGENS—substances that hamper the production of thyroid hormones by the thyroid gland. This can cause an enlargement of the gland (goiter) in an attempt by the body to compensate for the reduced hormone production by increasing the amount of tissue available. However, people with healthy thyroids would have to eat a very large amount of these vegetables before they would have any kind of problem. This is only of concern for those with sluggish thyroid glands. Goitrogens break down when the vegetable is heated and so anyone can eat as much of the cooked vegetable as they want.

CAVIAR

Serving Size: 1 ounce (sturgeon, granular)
Rating: ★

CALORIES: 74
CHOLESTEROL: 75 mg
FAT: 6 grams
SODIUM: 624 mg (Your maximum daily allowance is 300 mg!)
IRON: 18%
PHOSPHORUS: 10%
POTASSIUM: 51 mg
PROTEIN: 17%

GOOD POINTS

Caviar is low in calories, a good source of protein and iron, and contains significant amounts of calcium, phosphorus, and potassium.

Caviar is very high in artery-clogging cholesterol, and sodium, making it a bad choice for anyone in a high risk group for a heart attack. It also contains significant amounts of a substance called TYRAMINE, which can be very dangerous when consumed by someone who is on monoamine oxidase inhibitors (MAOI's), a group of antidepressant medications. Fish is sometimes the cause of ALLERGIC SYMPTOMS such as stomach upset, hives, and swelling of the face, lips, and eyes.

CEREAL, CORN FLAKES

Serving Size: 1 cup
Rating: ★★

CALORIES: 103
FAT: 1 gram
SODIUM: 325 mg
B COMPLEX VITAMINS: 33% for B1, 26% for B2, 29% for B3
COMPLEX CARBOHYDRATE: 24 grams
FIBER: 3 grams

GOOD POINTS

Corn flakes are an excellent source of the B vitamins, giving you energy, healthy eyes, skin and tissues. They also contain a significant amount of fiber, to prevent digestive problems.

BAD POINTS

This type of breakfast cereal is high in sodium, and contains a moderate amount of calories. It also contains a substance called GLUTEN which can cause an upset digestive system, anemia, weight loss, bone pain, skin problems, and water retention in people with a condition known as celiac disease.

CEREAL, OATMEAL OR ROLLED OATS

Serving Size: 1 cup (cooked)
Rating: ★★★

CALORIES: 132

FAT: 2 grams

B COMPLEX VITAMINS: 11% for B1, 5% for folic acid

COMPLEX CARBOHYDRATE: 24 grams

FIBER: 2.3 grams; some of it is in the form of pectin, which lowers blood cholesterol

IRON: 8%

MAGNESIUM: 9%

PHOSPHORUS: 13%

POTASSIUM: 5%

PROTEIN: 6%

ZINC: 5%

GOOD POINTS

The best choice for a breakfast cereal! Oatmeal or oat cereal contains a good amount of fiber and of a type that includes pectin, known to lower blood cholesterol levels. It also contains significant quantities of protein, potassium, magnesium, phosphorus, iron, zinc, vitamin B1, and folic acid.

BAD POINTS

Unfortunately, few things are perfect. Oatmeal is quite high in calories. It also contains a substance called GLUTEN which can cause an upset digestive system, anemia, weight loss, bone pain, skin problems, and water retention in people with a condition known as celiac disease.

CEREAL, RICE-BASED
Serving Size: 1 cup
Rating: ★★

CALORIES: 104

FAT: 0.2 grams

SODIUM: 310

B COMPLEX VITAMINS: 43% for B1, 28% for B2, 34% for B3

COMPLEX CARBOHYDRATE: 22 grams

FIBER: 4.3 grams

GOOD POINTS
Rice cereals are an excellent source of the B vitamins, for energy as well as healthy skin, eyes, and body tissues. They also contain good amounts of fiber that can keep your digestive system regular and disease-free.

BAD POINTS
Rice cereals are high in sodium and not particularly low in calories either.

CEREAL, SHREDDED WHEAT
Serving Size: 1 ounce
Rating: ★★

CALORIES: 90

FAT: 0.5 grams

B COMPLEX VITAMINS: 5% for B1, 6% for B3, 13% for B6

COMPLEX CARBOHYDRATE: 19 grams

COPPER: 19%

FIBER: 3.4 grams

IRON: 7%

MAGNESIUM: 9%

PHOSPHORUS: 10%

POTASSIUM: 92 mg

PROTEIN: 3 grams

GOOD POINTS

Shredded wheat contains some of the B vitamins, protein, fiber, potassium, magnesium, copper, phosphorus, and iron. Although it is not exactly low in calories, it contains less then the other types of breakfast cereal—but then again, some other types have more nutrients, as well.

BAD POINTS

It also contains a substance called GLUTEN which can cause an upset digestive system, anemia, weight loss, bone pain, skin problems, and water retention in people with a condition known as celiac disease.

CHEESE, AMERICAN

Serving Size: 1 ounce
Rating: ★

CALORIES: 106

CHOLESTEROL: 27

FAT: 9 grams

SODIUM: 406 mg

VITAMIN A: 8%

VITAMIN B2: 6%

CALCIUM: 17%

PHOSPHORUS: 21%

PROTEIN: 14%

ZINC: 40%

GOOD POINTS

American cheese is good for healthy skin and hair, is a fine source of protein, and is one of the best dietary sources of calcium. Since calcium is absorbed better from milk and dairy products than from any other food or supplement, cheese contributes to the development of stronger teeth and bones. Strong bones mean a reduced chance of developing osteoporosis in later life. American cheese also contains good quantities of vitamins A and B2, phosphorus and almost half your daily requirement for zinc.

BAD POINTS

This is not a food for dieters, because of its high calorie content. It is high in fat—most of it is the unpleasant form of saturated fat and cholesterol, which can raise your blood cholesterol levels and increase your risk of getting a heart attack or stroke. It is also high in sodium, which can increase your blood pressure or cause water retention (bloating) in susceptible people.

LACTOSE INTOLERANCE affects as many as two thirds of American adults. These people lack the enzyme lactase, which is needed to break down milk sugar (lactose). As a result, when they eat dairy products, the lactose passes through the digestive system where it is broken down by bacteria instead, causing FLATULENCE (gas), bloating, and diarrhea.

CHEESE, CHEDDAR

Serving Size: 1 ounce
Rating: ★★

CALORIES: 114
FAT: 9.4 ounces
VITAMIN A: 6%
VITAMIN B2: 6%
CALCIUM: 20%
PHOSPHORUS: 15%
PROTEIN: 16%

GOOD POINTS
Dairy products are the best source of calcium in our diets, which keeps our teeth and bones healthy. (They contain an ideal ratio of calcium to phosphorus for maximum calcium absorption.) Cheese is also a good source of protein and contains vitamin A and B2.

BAD POINTS
Before you add a slice of cheddar to your burger, you might want to consider this. It is high in saturated fat, high in sodium and high in calories. Aged cheddar also contains a significant amount of TYRAMINE, and therefore could present a problem to anyone taking the type of antidepressant medica-

tions known as monoamine oxidase inhibitors (MAOI's).

LACTOSE INTOLERANCE affects as many as two thirds of all adults, people who don't have an enzyme called lactase in their bodies, which is needed to break down milk sugar (lactose). As a result, when they eat dairy products, the lactose passes through the digestive system where it is broken down by bacteria instead, causing flatulence, bloating, and diarrhea.

CHEESE, COTTAGE
(CREAMED)

Serving Size: 1 cup
Rating: ★★

CALORIES: 217

CHOLESTEROL: 31 mg

FAT: 9.5 grams

SIMPLE CARBOHYDRATE: 5.6 grams

SODIUM: 850 mg

VITAMIN A: 7%

B COMPLEX VITAMINS: 20% for B2, 7% for B6, 22% for B12, and 7% for folic acid

CALCIUM: 13%

PHOSPHORUS: 28%

POTASSIUM: 177 mg

PROTEIN: 58%

GOOD POINTS
Cottage cheese is an excellent source of high quality protein, necessary for the growth and maintenance of every tissue in your body. It also contains substantial amounts of the B complex vitamins (especially B12, needed for blood formation and a healthy nervous system), calcium phosphorus, and potassium, as well as some vitamin A.

BAD POINTS
Cottage cheese is high in calories, sodium, saturated fat and cholesterol—making it a poor choice for people who are watching their weight, salt intake,

and/or their arteries! It also contains simple carbohydrate in the form of LACTOSE, which could cause digestive upsets in people with lactose intolerance. Many people are allergic to the protein in milk, which causes symptoms similar to those found with lactose intolerance, such as flatulence, bloating and diarrhea.

CHEESE, COTTAGE
(1% FAT)

Serving Size: 1 cup
Rating: ★★★

CALORIES: 164
CHOLESTEROL: 10 mg
FAT: 2.3 grams
SIMPLE CARBOHYDRATE: 6.2 grams
SODIUM: 918 mg
B COMPLEX VITAMINS: 22% for B2, 8% for B6, 24% for B12, and 7% for folic acid
CALCIUM: 14%
PHOSPHORUS: 30%
POTASSIUM: 193 mg
PROTEIN: 62%

GOOD POINTS

1% fat cottage cheese is a much better food choice than the regular creamed variety. It is still an excellent source of protein (needed for all tissue growth and maintenance), B complex vitamins (especially B12, for blood formation and a healthy nervous system), and a good source of calcium, phosphorus, and potassium. The difference here is that it is lower in fat and cholesterol, containing less then one third the amount found in creamed cottage cheese. However, it is still relatively high in calories and so not a great dieting choice.

BAD POINTS

It is still quite high in calories and can be ever higher in sodium than creamed cottage cheese (unless otherwise indicated on the product). It also contains a small amount of fat and cholesterol.

Cottage cheese has simple carbohydrate in the form of **LACTOSE**, which could cause digestive upsets in people with lactose intolerance. Many people are allergic to the protein in milk, which causes symptoms similar to those found with lactose intolerance, such as flatulence, bloating, and diarrhea.

CHEESE, MOZZARELLA

Serving Size: 1 ounce
Rating: ★★

CALORIES: 80
CHOLESTEROL: 22 mg
FAT: 8.1 grams
SODIUM: 106 mg
VITAMIN A: 5%
CALCIUM: 15%
VITAMIN D: 5%
IODINE: 81%
PHOSPHORUS: 11%
PROTEIN: 12%

GOOD POINTS

This type of stringy cheese is an excellent source of iodine. Since it's a milk product, it is also one of the best dietary sources of calcium. It contains good amounts of protein and phosphorus, along with a little bit of vitamins A and D.

BAD POINTS

Although it has 25% fewer calories then most other hard cheeses, it is still not an ideal food for dieters. It also contains quite a lot of fat, (much of it saturated), sodium and cholesterol, making it bad for heart and blood pressure-watchers.

Some people don't have an enzyme called lactase in their bodies, which is needed to break down milk sugar (lactose). As a result, when they eat dairy products, the lactose passes through the digestive system where it is broken down by bacteria instead, causing flatulence, bloating and diarrhea. Allergies to the protein in milk, causing symptoms similar to those of lactose intolerance, also affect many people.

Mozzarella cheese also contains significant amounts of a substance called TYRAMINE, which can be very dangerous when consumed by someone who is taking monoamine oxidase inhibitors (MAOI's), a group of antidepressant medications.

CHEESE, SWISS

Serving Size: 1 ounce (1-2 slices)
Rating: ★★

CALORIES: 107
CHOLESTEROL: 26 mg
FAT: 7.8 grams
SODIUM: 74 mg
B COMPLEX VITAMINS: 6% for B2, 8% for B12
CALCIUM: 27%
PHOSPHORUS: 17%
PROTEIN: 18%
ZINC: 7%

GOOD POINTS
Swiss cheese is a very good source of calcium, needed to build bones and teeth and to keep bones strong. It is also a good source of protein and phosphorus, and contains some B vitamins and zinc.

BAD POINTS
It's high in calories and fat (mainly saturated), as well as cholesterol. It also contains a little sodium. All in all, it's not the best choice for health and weight-conscious eaters.

Some people don't have an enzyme called lactase in their bodies, which is needed to break down milk sugar (lactose). As a result, when they eat dairy products, the lactose passes through the digestive system where it is broken down by bacteria instead, causing flatulence, bloating, and diarrhea. Allergies to the protein in milk products, causing symptoms similar to those of lactose intolerance, also affect many people.

Cheesecake

Serving Size: 1 piece
Rating: ★

CALORIES: 257
FAT: 16.3 grams
COMPLEX CARBOHYDRATE: Approx. 15 grams
SIMPLE CARBOHYDRATE: Approx. 9 grams
SODIUM: 189 mg
B COMPLEX VITAMINS: 6% for B2, 7% for B12
PHOSPHORUS: 8%
POTASSIUM: 83 mg
PROTEIN: 10%

GOOD POINTS
Cheesecake contains significant amounts of protein, potassium, phosphorus, and vitamins B2 and B12. However, because of the bad points listed below it is not a good source for any of these nutrients.

BAD POINTS
Cheesecake is extremely high in calories, saturated fat, and sodium, making it bad for dieters, for those on salt-restricted diets, and for people who need to lower their blood cholesterol levels. It also contains simple carbohydrate, which contributes to tooth decay, as well as a substance called GLUTEN that can cause an upset digestive system, anemia, weight loss, bone pain, skin problems, and water retention in people with a condition known as celiac disease.

CHERRIES

Serving Size: 10 cherries (sweet, raw)
Rating: ★

CALORIES: 49
FAT: 0.7 grams
SIMPLE CARBOHYDRATE: 11.3 grams
VITAMIN C: 12%
CALORIES: 49
POTASSIUM: 152 mg
FAT: 0.7 grams

GOOD POINTS
Cherries are a good source of vitamin C, an "anti-cancer" nutrient that maintains the health of your immune system. They also contain potassium, and happily, relatively few calories. For a special sweet treat while you're on that strict diet, try nibbling a few cherries.

BAD POINTS
All of the carbohydrate found in cherries is in the form of simple sugars, which can cause tooth decay.

MARASCHINO CHERRIES

Serving Size: 2 medium
Rating: Nope, no stars

CALORIES: 19
FAT: 0.2 grams

GOOD POINTS
None, except for a low fat content

BAD POINTS
These pretty little garnishes contain 19 empty calories. Some hyperactive children may be sensitive to the RED DYES used to color them.

CHEWING GUM

Serving Size: 1 stick
Rating: Sorry, no stars

CALORIES: 19
FAT: None
SIMPLE CARBOHYDRATE: 4.6 grams

GOOD POINTS
None, besides its negligible fat content.

BAD POINTS
Chewing gum is full of simple sugars, which can cause tooth decay. Sugar-free gum does not have this drawback and also contains about half as many calories.

CHICKEN
(ROASTED)

Serving Size: 3.5 ounces
Rating:★★★

CALORIES (WITH SKIN): 239 (WITHOUT SKIN): 190
CHOLESTEROL: 88 mg
FAT: 14 grams (about 7 grams if skin is removed)
SODIUM: 82 mg
B COMPLEX VITAMINS: 10% for B2, 43% for B3, 23% for B6, 5% for B12, and 10% for pantothenic acid
IRON: 7%
MAGNESIUM: 6%
PHOSPHORUS: 18%
POTASSIUM: 223 mg
PROTEIN: 61%
ZINC: 10%

GOOD POINTS
Chicken is an excellent source of many beneficial nutrients. It provides good quality protein and lots of the B complex vitamins, as well as respectable amounts

of phosphorus, magnesium, iron, zinc, and potassium. It can be served in a wide variety of ways, hot or cold, and for many people with gastrointestinal problems, it is an easy food to digest. For a main course, it is also not especially high in calories, although weight watchers should always take off the skin.

BAD POINTS

Chicken contains quite a bit of fat, although this is equally divided into saturated and unsaturated fat. Removing the skin cuts down the fat content by half, but makes no difference to its significant cholesterol content. Why then do people feel that chicken is somehow better for you than beef? Although chicken and lean beef contain about the same amounts of fat and cholesterol, the fat in the beef is mainly all saturated as opposed to the nice balance found in chicken. (When saturated and polyunsaturated are in this type of balance, the fat does not raise blood cholesterol levels. However, the cholesterol found in the food still does.)

Chicken also contains some sodium and so should not be eaten to excess by those on strict salt-free diets.

CHOCOLATE
(MILK CHOCOLATE)

Serving Size: 1 ounce (1 standard bar)
Rating: 1/2★

CALORIES: 148
FAT: 8.5 grams
SIMPLE CARBOHYDRATE: 16.6 grams
CALCIUM: 6%
PHOSPHORUS: 7%
POTASSIUM: 117.6 mg

GOOD POINTS

Well, it may not be great for you, but it is delicious, isn't it? Chocolate does contain a respectable amount of calcium and phosphorus and a good amount of potassium. Plain chocolate contains less of these nutrients.

BAD POINTS

The piece of chocolate you're craving is high in simple sugars, calories, and contains significant amounts of saturated fat. However, this news is not quite as bad as it sounds because the fat in chocolate forms a film on the teeth that protects it from the decay-causing nature of the sugar.

Many people show ALLERGIC REACTIONS to chocolate, and it also contains TYRAMINE, which will be a problem for anyone taking the type of antidepressant drugs known as monoamine oxidase inhibitors (MAOIs).

Chocolate is rich in CAFFEINE and caffeine-like compounds so don't eat too much of it before bedtime.

CHOCOLATE CAKE

Serving Size: 1 piece
Rating:★

CALORIES: 227

FAT: 11.3 grams

SIMPLE CARBOHYDRATE: approx. 20

SODIUM: 160 mg

VITAMIN B2: 7%

CALCIUM: 7%

IRON: 6%

MAGNESIUM: 6%

PHOSPHORUS: 8%

POTASSIUM: 95 mg

PROTEIN: 5%

GOOD POINTS

Chocolate cake contains small but effective amounts of several essential nutrients—protein, vitamin B2, calcium, phosphorus, magnesium, iron, and potassium—but these are really not much to get in exchange for all those calories!

BAD POINTS

This food is very high in calories, which should come as no surprise. It also contains a lot of fat (of the bad, cholesterol-raising saturated variety), as well as simple carbohydrate, which can cause tooth decay. One good thing is that the fat from the cocoa beans in chocolate coats the teeth and forms a protective barrier against the bacteria that cause tooth decay.

Chocolate cake is also high in sodium, and so off the list for those on salt-restricted diets. People may also suffer from ALLERGIC REACTIONS to the chocolate, and it contains TYRAMINE, which doesn't combine well with the monoamine oxidase inhibitor (MAOI) class of drug. Since it contains caffeine, it is not an ideal bedtime snack.

CHOCOLATE MILK

Serving Size: 1 cup
Rating: ★★★

CALORIES: 208

CHOLESTEROL: 30 mg

FAT: 8.5 grams

SIMPLE CARBOHYDRATE: 25.9 grams

B COMPLEX VITAMINS: 6% for B1, 24% for B2, 5% for B6, 14% for B12 and 7% for pantothenic acid

CALCIUM: 28%

COPPER: 7%

VITAMIN D: 10%

MAGNESIUM: 8%

PHOSPHORUS: 25%

POTASSIUM: 417 mg

PROTEIN: 17%

ZINC: 5%

GOOD POINTS

Chocolate milk is an excellent source of calcium (for strong bones and teeth, and many other body functions), phosphorus (for bones, teeth, enzymes, and new cells), and B12 (for energy, healthy tissues, good skin and eyes). It also contains healthy amounts of vitamins A, B1, B6, B12, pantothenic acid, D, protein, magnesium, copper, potassium, and zinc.

BAD POINTS

While it contains a lot of calories, 1% and 2% fat chocolate milks have significantly less (50 and 29 calories less, respectively). It is also high in saturated fat and cholesterol and so not advised for anyone on a cholesterol-restricted diet (1% fat milk has about half as much, but 2% has about the same). Chocolate milk also contains a lot of simple sugars, but the fat in the milk helps to guard against tooth decay. It is high in sodium and therefore off limits for those on salt-restricted diets.

Many people may be ALLERGIC to the chocolate. Since it contains caffeine it should not be drunk before bedtime, and it also has a substance called TYRAMINE, which does not combine well with the class of drugs known as MAOI's (monoamine oxidase inhibitors). (While all forms of chocolate contain a substance called OXALIC ACID that reduces calcium absorption slightly, chocolate milk is still a good source of the mineral.)

CLAMS

Serving Size: 4 large
Rating:★★★

CALORIES: 82
CHOLESTEROL: 65 mg
FAT: 0.3 grams
B COMPLEX VITAMINS: 7% for B1, 12% for B2, 7% for B3
VITAMIN C: 18%
CALCIUM: 8%
CALORIES: 82
IODINE: 10%
IRON: 30%
PHOSPHORUS: 18%
POTASSIUM: 235 mg
PROTEIN: 31%
FAT: 0.3 grams

GOOD POINTS

Clams are a concentrated, low-calorie source of good quality protein and one of the best dietary sources of well-absorbed iron. Protein is essential for building and repairing all tissues in the body, as well as for protecting against infection. Iron is needed for healthy blood and muscles, and is a part of many enzymes and proteins. The refreshing clam appetizer or main dish also contains potassium, phosphorus, iodine, calcium, and vitamins B1, B2, B3, and C.

BAD POINTS
Clams are high in cholesterol. Shellfish are also one of the food types most often found to be a cause of ALLERGIC REACTIONS. They can transmit INFECTIOUS DISEASES including hepatitis B, worms, and parasites and so should always be cooked thoroughly—quick steaming is NOT enough. Shellfish also pick up microorganisms from the water that can cause an upset stomach. From July through October, they can pick up organisms called DINOFLAGELLATES that float on the surface of the Atlantic and Pacific ocean off the coast and cause the "red tide." These may produce a nervous system poison that cannot be destroyed by cooking.

COCKTAILS

Serving Size: 1 cocktail (3.5 fluid ounces)
Rating: Nope, no stars

CALORIES: 160
FAT: none, except for pina coladas, which can contain as much as 16 grams!

GOOD POINTS
None, except for a lack of fat.

BAD POINTS
Cocktails, like martinis and manhattans, are high in calories. Not only does alcohol provide no essential nutrients but it actually DEPLETES THE BODY of vitamins A, B1, B2, B6, D, folic acid, calcium, magnesium, zinc, and glucose.

COCONUT

Serving Size: 1 ounce
Rating: No stars

CALORIES: 98
FAT: 10 grams
FIBER: 3.8 grams
POTASSIUM: 167 mg

GOOD POINTS

Coconut is a good source of non-pectin fiber to help the digestive system, as well as potassium (for muscle function, maintenance of a correct fluid balance in the body, a healthy nervous system, and to help the body get energy from food). The reason it is a "no-star" food is explained by its drawbacks.

BAD POINTS

Coconut is the most concentrated source of saturated fat in our food supply. Although it does not contain cholesterol, it should never be included on a cholesterol-lowering diet. This high fat content of course makes it a high calorie food as well, Nuts, including coconut, can cause ALLERGIC REACTIONS in susceptible people.

COD (BROILED)

Serving Size: 3.5 ounces
Rating:★★★★

CALORIES: 83
FAT: 0.7 grams
SODIUM: 100 mg
B COMPLEX VITAMINS: 6% for B1, 5% for B2, 11% for B3, 19% for B6 and 50% for B12
IODINE: 10%
MAGNESIUM: 5%
PHOSPHORUS: 24%
POTASSIUM: 360 mg
PROTEIN: 41%

GOOD POINTS

Cod is an excellent source of good quality protein and the B complex vitamins (especially B12, needed for a healthy nervous system and the formation of red blood cells). In addition it is low in calories and contains potassium, magnesium, phosphorus, and iodine (for a healthy thyroid gland).

BAD POINTS

Cod contains significant amounts of sodium. Fish is sometimes the cause of ALLERGIC SYMPTOMS such as stomach upset, hives, and swelling of the face, lips and eyes.

COD LIVER OIL

Serving Size: 1 teaspoon
Rating:★★

CALORIES: 135
FAT: 15 grams
VITAMIN A: 54%
VITAMIN D: 300%
VITAMIN E: 15%
IODINE: 100%

GOOD POINTS

Cod liver oil, not normally the most popular of foods, is one of the richest sources of vitamin A for healthy skin, eyes, teeth, hair, bones, glands, and effective immune system. It is also the richest dietary source of vitamin D (essential for calcium absorption and hence strong bones and teeth), and contains the whole RDA for iodine (essential for the production of thyroid hormone), as well as some vitamin E.

BAD POINTS

It contains significant amounts of fat, but of a kind known as the omega-3 fatty acids, which tend to lower blood cholesterol levels. However, eating any sort of fat seems to raise your risk of getting breast, uterine, endometrial, ovarian, prostate, and colon cancer. It is also high in calories.

Too much vitamin D is not good for you, because it can cause CALCIUM DEPOSITS in the body, including in the arteries. Therefore, you should not make a habit of eating this food product too often.

COFFEE

Serving Size: 1 cup (6 fluid ounces)
Rating: Sorry, no stars

CALORIES: 3
FAT: none
VITAMIN B3: 7%
POTASSIUM: 117 mg

GOOD POINTS
The drink that most of us hold under our noses each morning contains only a little vitamin B3 and some potassium. But it doesn't have many calories, either.

BAD POINTS
Coffee stimulates ACID SECRETION IN THE STOMACH (this holds true for both regular and decaffeinated). One cup of brewed coffee contains over 100 mg of caffeine (60 mg for instant, 150 mg for drip, and 5 mg for decaffeinated). CAFFEINE impairs the body's absorption of iron when taken with foods rich in iron, such as red meats and shellfish. This could be a problem for those with a poor iron status, such as women who menstruate heavily, the elderly, and some teenagers. Caffeine has also be implicated in other areas which are more controversial, such as painful breasts and PMS.

COLE SLAW

Serving Size: 1 cup
Rating:★

CALORIES: 173
FAT: 16.8 grams
SODIUM: 144 mg
VITAMIN C: 58%
CALCIUM: 5%
FIBER: 0.8 grams
POTASSIUM: 239 mg

GOOD POINTS

Cole slaw, the "deli" side dish, is rich in vitamin C (for healthy muscles, blood vessels, bones, teeth, and gums, and needed by those weak in the vitamin, such as women on oral contraceptives and smokers). It also contains some calcium, fiber, and potassium.

BAD POINTS

It is high in calories and fat. The kind of fat is dependant on the type of mayonnaise used to make it, but it is usually polyunsaturated (which lowers blood cholesterol but can increase your risk of getting certain types of cancers). It also contains quite a lot of sodium, and so is not recommended for those on salt-restricted diets.

COLLARD GREENS

Serving Size: 1/2 cup (cooked)
Rating:★★★★

CALORIES: 29
FAT: 0.4 grams
VITAMIN A: 108%
B COMPLEX VITAMINS: 9% for B1, 12% for B2, 7% for B3
VITAMIN C: 77%
CALCIUM: 15%
FIBER: 0.8 mg
POTASSIUM: 234 mg

GOOD POINTS

While it is more popular in some areas of the country than others, this low-calorie vegetable is an excellent source of vitamin A (as carotene, which protects against cancers of the digestive and respiratory tract). It is also rich in vitamin C and calcium, and contains good amounts of vitamins B1, B2, B3, and potassium and fiber.

BAD POINTS

Collard greens contain NITRATES, which are converted in the body into NITRITES and NITROSAMINES—potential carcinogens (cancer-causing agents). If the greens are fresh, this is not a problem, but if they are cooked and left standing for some time at room temperature, bacteria that convert nitrates to nitrites multiply and the level of nitrites rises significantly.

CONSOMMÉ

Serving Size: 1 cup
Rating: ★

CALORIES: 29
FAT: none
SODIUM: 637 mg
POTASSIUM: 153 mg
PROTEIN: 12%

GOOD POINTS

Consommé is low in calories (although its sodium content might make it a bad food for dieters) and surprisingly high in protein and potassium. It is a good choice for someone with diarrhea or nausea.

BAD POINTS

This soup is very high in sodium and so not good for people on salt-restricted diets, or for dieters who are susceptible to water retention.

COOKIES, CHOCOLATE CHIP

Serving Size: 1 small
Rating: No stars

CALORIES: 46
FAT: 2.7 grams
SIMPLE CARBOHYDRATE: 6.4 grams

GOOD POINTS
None.

BAD POINTS
Much as we hate to say it, the truth is that chocolate chip cookies are nothing but empty calories—and lots of them at that! They contain no essential nutrients in meaningful amounts but they do contain sugar (which makes your teeth susceptible to decay) and some fat. In addition, many people are ALLERGIC to chocolate. Cookies also contain a substance called GLUTEN which can cause an upset digestive system, anemia, weight loss, bone pain, skin problems, and water retention in people with a condition known as celiac disease.

COOKIES, OATMEAL

Serving Size: 1 small
Rating: No stars

CALORIES: 62
FAT: 2.6 grams
SIMPLE CARBOHYDRATE: 8.9 grams

GOOD POINTS
None.

BAD POINTS
Oatmeal cookies may sound better for you than the other types but they're not. They offer up a significant number of calories, simple sugars (which can cause tooth decay), and some fat, but only insignif-

icant amounts of essential nutrients. In addition, they contain a substance called GLUTEN which can cause an upset digestive system, anemia, weight loss, bone pain, skin problems, and water retention in people with a condition known as celiac disease.

COOKIES, WAFERS

Serving Size: 2 wafers
Rating: No stars

CALORIES: 62
FAT: 2.6 grams
SIMPLE CARBOHYDRATE: 8.9 grams

GOOD POINTS
None.

BAD POINTS
Wafers can't give you any meaningful quantities of essential nutrients, but they do offer a significant amount of calories, simple sugars (that promote tooth decay), and some fat. In addition, they contain a substance called GLUTEN which can cause an upset digestive system, anemia, weight loss, bone pain, skin problems, and water retention in people with a condition known as celiac disease.

CORDIALS AND LIQUEURS

Serving Size: 1 fluid ounce
Rating: Sorry, no stars

CALORIES: 97
FAT: most contain 0.1 grams, except for coffee with cream, which contains about 8 grams
SIMPLE CARBOHYDRATE: 11.5 grams

GOOD POINTS
None.

These drinks are high in calories but not in essential nutrients. They also contain simple sugars, which can cause tooth decay. To make matters even worse, 54% proof liqueurs and cordials are 22.1% alcohol, and alcohol DEPLETES THE BODY of vitamins A, B1, B2, B6, D, folic acid, calcium, magnesium, zinc, and glucose.

CORN ON THE COB

Serving Size: 4-inch ear
Rating: ★★★

CALORIES: 100
FAT: 1 gram
VITAMIN A: 8%
B COMPLEX VITAMINS: 8% for B1, 6% for B2
VITAMIN C: 25%
COMPLEX CARBOHYDRATE: 21 grams
FIBER: 0.7 grams; some of it is in the form of pectin, which lowers blood cholesterol
PHOSPHORUS: 9%
POTASSIUM: 196 mg
PROTEIN: 5%

GOOD POINTS

Corn is a good source of vitamin A, in the form of carotene, and vitamin C, both of which help protect you from cancers of the respiratory and gastrointestinal tracts. It also contains generous helpings of the B complex vitamins, potassium, and phosphorus, and has some fiber and protein. This vegetable is a healthy, sweet, and fun choice for a side dish, provided you don't smother it with heaps of butter!

BAD POINTS

Corn on the cob is relatively high in calories, and so not the best vegetable for dieters. ALLERGIES to corn are also common.

CRAB

Serving Size: 3.5 ounces
Rating:★★★

CALORIES: 93
CHOLESTEROL: 100 mg
FAT: 1.9 grams
SODIUM: 370 mg
VITAMIN A: 43%
B COMPLEX VITAMINS: 11% for B1, 9% for B2, 14% for B3, 18% for B6, and 5% for folic acid
IODINE: 10%
IRON: 5%
MAGNESIUM: 12%
PHOSPHORUS: 18%
POTASSIUM: 270 mg
PROTEIN: 38%
ZINC: 37%

GOOD POINTS

Toss some crab into that seafood salad! It's high in vitamin A, protein, and zinc—all needed for a healthy immune system, hair and skin. It's also a good source of the B vitamins, iron, iodine, phosphorus, magnesium, and potassium, and is low in calories.

BAD POINTS

But don't put too much crab in the salad! It's high in cholesterol, although most of the rest of the fat it contains is rich in the omega-3 fatty acids which help to reduce the cholesterol-raising effect. However, you should remember that the latest recommendations advise against eating more than 300 mg of cholesterol per day. Crab is high in sodium, so it should be off the salt-watchers diet. Shellfish are also common causes of ALLERGIC SYMPTOMS, and they can be contaminated with CHOLERA or HEPATITIS B. Be sure to clean and cook them thoroughly.

CRACKER

Serving Size: 2
Rating:★

CALORIES: 44
FAT: 1.6 grams
SODIUM: 61 mg
COMPLEX CARBOHYDRATE: approx. 6 grams

GOOD POINTS

Crackers are low in calories and fat but provide very little in the way of nutrients. They are good to take to prevent further nausea after vomiting.

BAD POINTS

They contain some fat and sodium, and are often made from wheat flour, which contains a substance called GLUTEN and can cause an upset digestive system, anemia, weight loss, bone pain, skin problems, and water retention in people with a condition known as celiac disease.

CRANBERRIES

Serving Size: 1 cup
Rating:★★

CALORIES: 46
FAT: 0.2 grams
SIMPLE CARBOHYDRATES: 12.1 grams
VITAMIN C: 22%
FIBER: 1.1 grams
POTASSIUM: 67 mg

GOOD POINTS

Cranberries are a good source of vitamin C and contain some potassium and fiber. They are also low in calories. The C content is important for healthy teeth, gums, blood vessels, bones and as protection against disease. It also aids in iron absorption, and may help protect you against cancer.

BAD POINTS

Cranberries contain quite a lot of simple sugar which can encourage the bacteria that cause tooth decay.

CREAM, HALF AND HALF

Serving Size: 1 tablespoon
Rating: No stars

CALORIES: 20
CHOLESTEROL: 6 mg
FAT: 1.7 grams

GOOD POINT
None.

BAD POINTS

Cream is high in calories and relatively high in fat and cholesterol (although half and half is better than full cream).

Some people don't have an enzyme called **LACTASE** in their bodies, which is needed to break down milk sugar (lactose). As a result, when they eat dairy products, the lactose passes through the digestive system where it is broken down by bacteria instead, causing flatulence, bloating, and diarrhea. Allergies to the protein in milk, causing symptoms similar to those of lactose intolerance, also affect many people.

CREAM, HEAVY WHIPPING

Serving Size: 1 tablespoon
Rating: No stars

CALORIES: 52
CHOLESTEROL: 21 mg
FAT: 5.6 grams

GOOD POINTS
None.

BAD POINTS

This food is high in calories, saturated fat and cholesterol, and is best avoided by everybody, but especially by those who are heart-smart.

Some people don't have an enzyme called LACTASE in their bodies, which is needed to break down milk sugar (lactose). As a result, when they eat dairy products, the lactose passes through the digestive system where it is broken down by bacteria instead, causing flatulence, bloating, and diarrhea. Allergies to the protein in milk, causing symptoms similar to those of lactose intolerance, also affect many people.

CREAM, LIGHT (FOR COFFEE)

Serving Size: 1 tablespoon
Rating: No stars

CALORIES: 29
CHOLESTEROL: 10 mg
FAT: 2.9 grams

GOOD POINTS
None.

BAD POINTS

This type of cream is also high in calories and relatively high in cholesterol and saturated fat.

Some people don't have an enzyme called LACTASE in their bodies, which is needed to break down milk sugar (lactose). As a result, when they eat dairy products, the lactose passes through the digestive system where it is broken down by bacteria instead, causing flatulence, bloating, and diarrhea. Allergies to the protein in milk, causing symptoms similar to those of lactose intolerance, also affect many people.

CREAM (SOUR)

Serving Size: 1 tablespoon
Rating: Nope, no stars

CALORIES: 26
CHOLESTEROL: 5 mg
FAT: 2.5 grams

GOOD POINTS
None.

BAD POINTS
Although people tend to think of sour cream as being better for you than the other creams, it really isn't. It's high in calories, and relatively high in cholesterol and saturated fat.

Some people don't have an enzyme called LACTASE in their bodies, which is needed to break down milk sugar (lactose). As a result, when they eat dairy products, the lactose passes through the digestive system where it is broken down by bacteria instead, causing flatulence, bloating, and diarrhea. Allergies to the protein in milk, causing symptoms similar to those of lactose intolerance, also affect many people.

CREAM CHEESE

Serving Size: 2 tablespoons
Rating: ★

CALORIES: 99
CHOLESTEROL: 31 mg
FAT: 9.9 grams
SODIUM: 84 mg
VITAMIN A: 8%
PROTEIN: 34%

GOOD POINTS
Cream cheese contains a lot of good quality protein, needed for the growth and maintenance of all the tissues in your body as well as a strong immune

system. It also contains a significant amount of vitamin A.

BAD POINTS
It is very high in calories, saturated fat, and cholesterol and so is not a good food for anyone trying to lose weight or lower blood cholesterol levels. It also has significant amounts of sodium.

Some people don't have an enzyme called LACTASE in their bodies, which is needed to break down milk sugar (lactose). As a result, when they eat dairy products, the lactose passes through the digestive system where it is broken down by bacteria instead, causing flatulence, bloating and diarrhea. Allergies to the protein in milk, causing symptoms similar to those of lactose intolerance, also affect many people.

CUCUMBER
Serving Size: ¹/₂ cucumber
Rating: ★★

CALORIES: 8
FAT: 0.1 grams
VITAMIN C: 13%
POTASSIUM: 80 mg

GOOD POINTS
This vegetable contains a significant amount of vitamin C, important for healthy teeth, gums, blood vessels, bones and as protection against disease (C also aids in iron absorption, and may help protect you against cancer.) Cucumbers have significant quantities of potassium, and are extremely low in calories, as well. Salads full of greens like cucumbers make great fillers for dieters.

BAD POINTS
Cucumbers can cause FLATULENCE in some people.

CUSTARD

Serving Size: 1/2 cup
Rating: ★

CALORIES: 161
CHOLESTEROL: 80 mg
FAT: 5.4 grams
SIMPLE CARBOHYDRATE: 22.9 grams
SODIUM: 219 mg
B COMPLEX VITAMINS: 5% for B1, 16% for B2, 12% for B12, and 8% for pantothenic acid
CALCIUM: 19%
MAGNESIUM: 6%
PHOSPHORUS: 17%
POTASSIUM: 254 mg
PROTEIN: 5.4 grams

GOOD POINTS

A good source of calcium, phosphorus and magnesium for healthy bones and teeth, it is also high in the B complex vitamins and potassium, and contains some protein as well.

BAD POINTS

Custard is high in calories, cholesterol, and has a significant amount of saturated fat. Obviously, it's off the menu for dieters and artery-watchers. It is also pretty high in sodium, which similarly makes it off limits for those who retain water and/or have high blood pressure. It contains lots of simple carbohydrate, which can promote tooth decay.

Some people don't have an enzyme called lactase in their bodies, which is needed to break down milk sugar (lactose). As a result, when they eat dairy products, the lactose passes through the digestive system where it is broken down by bacteria instead, causing flatulence, bloating and diarrhea. Allergies to the protein in milk, causing symptoms similar to those of lactose intolerance, also affect many people.

DATES

Serving Size: 10 dried
Rating: ★★

CALORIES: 228
FAT: 0.4 grams
SIMPLE CARBOHYDRATE: 60 grams
B COMPLEX VITAMINS: 5% for B1, 9% for B3, 8% for B6, and 7% for pantothenic acid.
COPPER: 10%
FIBER: 1.8 grams
IRON: 5%
MAGNESIUM: 7%
POTASSIUM: 541 mg

GOOD POINTS

Dates are a very good source of potassium—needed for proper muscle contractions (including those of the heart), for maintaining the correct fluid balance in the body, to help the transmission of nerve impulses, and for the release of energy from the carbohydrate and protein you eat. This sweet and rather exotic fruit also has significant amounts of the B complex vitamins, magnesium, iron, copper, and a little fiber.

BAD POINTS

Dates are extremely high in calories in the form of simple sugars. Since they are sticky, they deposit sugar on the teeth, providing an excellent breeding ground for the bacteria that cause tooth decay.

Dates are often treated with SULFITES to preserve them. Some people are allergic to these substances and could develop symptoms such as rashes, watery eyes and breathing problems.

DISTILLED SPIRITS
(GIN, RUM, VODKA, WHISKEY)

Serving Size: 1 fluid ounce
Rating: No stars

CALORIES: 65 to 100 (for 80 proof)
FAT: None

GOOD POINTS
None, except that they contain no fat.

BAD POINTS
Distilled spirits contain no essential nutrients but they are full of calories. The alcohol content DEPLETES THE BODY of vitamins A, B1, B2, B6, D, folic acid, calcium, magnesium, zinc, and glucose. As the "proof" (alcohol content) increases, the calorie content rises as well.

DOUGHNUT

Serving Size: 1
Rating: No stars

CALORIES: 105
FAT: 5.8 grams
COMPLEX CARBOHYDRATE: approx. 5–6 grams
SIMPLE CARBOHYDRATE: approx. 5–7 grams
SODIUM: 139 mg
PHOSPHORUS: 6%

GOOD POINTS
Doughnuts contain significant amounts of phosphorus (but not much else), which is needed for strong bones and teeth, for the release of energy from the food you eat, and for the formation of new cells and enzymes.

BAD POINTS
This poor breakfast or snack choice is extremely high in calories, and filled doughnuts are even higher than

plain ones (for example, the standard jelly doughnut contains 226 calories!). They are also high in fat (mainly saturated) and sodium, making them the wrong food for people with (or those who are trying to avoid) cardiovascular disease and blood pressure problems. They have substantial amounts of simple sugars, which can cause tooth decay.

In addition, they contain a substance called GLUTEN which can cause an upset digestive system, anemia, weight loss, bone pain, skin problems, and water retention in people with a condition known as celiac disease.

DUCK

Serving Size: 3.5 ounces
Rating: ★★

CALORIES: 339

CHOLESTEROL: 84 mg

FAT: 29 grams

SODIUM: 76 mg

B COMPLEX VITAMINS: 11% for B1, 16% for B2, 9% for B3, 9% for B6, 5% for B12, and 5% for pantothenic acid

COPPER: 14%

IRON: 15%

PHOSPHORUS: 15%

POTASSIUM: 210 mg

PROTEIN: 44%

ZINC: 15%

GOOD POINTS
Duck is a very good source of high quality protein, required for the growth and maintenance of all your body tissues. It is also rich in B vitamins, potassium, zinc, copper, iron, and phosphorus. A duck salad can be used as the basis of a gourmet-type lunch.

BAD POINTS
Duck is pretty high in calories if eaten with the skin; without the skin the calorie content drops by at least a third. It is also high in fat (mainly saturated),

sodium and cholesterol, and so not advised for people who need to eat heart-smart foods, or who are watching their salt intake.

EGGPLANT

Serving Size: ¹/₂ cup (cooked)
Rating: ★

CALORIES: 19
FAT: None
COMPLEX CARBOHYDRATE: 4 grams
FIBER: 0.9 grams
POTASSIUM: 150 mg

GOOD POINTS

This vegetable is very low in calories, and contains significant amounts of potassium, needed for proper muscle contractions (including those of the heart), for maintaining the correct fluid balance in the body, to help the transmission of nerve impulses, and for the release of energy from the carbohydrate and protein you eat. It also has a little fiber, and is a good, tasty side dish or basis for lasagna if you're watching your weight.

BAD POINTS

Eggplant contains a lot of NITRATES, which are converted in the body into NITRATES and NITROSAMINES—potential carcinogens (cancer-causing agents). If the eggplant is fresh, this is not a problem, but if it is cooked and left standing for some time at room temperature, bacteria that convert nitrates to nitrites multiply and the level of nitrites rises significantly. It also contains significant amounts of a substance called TYRAMINE, which can be very dangerous when consumed by someone who is taking monoamine oxidase inhibitors (MAOI's), a group of antidepressant medications.

EGGS

Serving Size: 1 large
Rating: ★★

CALORIES: 79

CHOLESTEROL: 274 (all in the yolk)

FAT: 5.6 grams

SODIUM: 69 mg

VITAMIN A: 5%

B COMPLEX VITAMINS: 9% for B2, 11% for B12, 6% for folic acid, and 9% for pantothenic acid

VITAMIN D: 9%

IRON: 6%

PHOSPHORUS: 9%

POTASSIUM: 65 mg

PROTEIN: 14%

GOOD POINTS
Eggs contain the best protein of any food in our diets, which is why they were traditionally fed to children (since protein is needed for the growth, maintenance, and repair of all body tissues). However, these days eggs don't have such a sterling name, mainly because of their cholesterol content. They do supply good amounts of the B vitamins, vitamins A and D, potassium, phosphorus, iron, and zinc, and believe it or not, they're relatively low in calories.

BAD POINTS
The most negative health aspect about eggs is, of course, their cholesterol content. The yolk contains 274 mg of cholesterol, which is about all of the stuff you're advised to eat in an entire day! Any more than that is believed to raise your risk of heart disease. They also contain significant amounts of fat and sodium (but if you leave out the yolk, eggs are actually a good food choice). Many people are ALLERGIC to eggs, and can develop symptoms such as itching and hives.

ENDIVE

Serving Size: 20 long leaves
Rating: ★★★★

CALORIES: 20
FAT: 0.2 grams
VITAMIN A: 66%
B COMPLEX VITAMINS: 8% for B2, 83% for folic acid
VITAMIN C: 17%
CALCIUM: 8%
COMPLEX CARBOHYDRATE: 4.1 grams
FIBER: 0.9 grams
IRON: 9%
PHOSPHORUS: 5%
POTASSIUM: 294 mg

GOOD POINTS
This new and popular addition to salads is one of the best foods in anyone's book! Endives are a superb source of vitamin A in the form of carotene, and folic acid. Vitamin A is needed for healthy skin, hair, and eyes, and helps protect the body from respiratory and gastrointestinal tract cancer. Folic acid is needed for the manufacture of all new cells in the body, including red blood cells; a deficiency in this vitamin is one of the main causes of anemia. But the good news doesn't stop there! Endives also contain vitamin C, vitamin B2, calcium, phosphorus, iron, potassium, and fiber, and are extremely low in calories.

BAD POINTS
None at all.

FIGS
(DRIED)

Serving Size: 3
Rating: ★★

CALORIES: 160
FAT: 0.7 grams
SIMPLE CARBOHYDRATE: 36 grams
VITAMIN B6: 6%

CALCIUM: 8%

COPPER: 9%

FIBER: 2.7 grams; some of it is in the form of pectin, which lowers blood cholesterol

IRON: 7%

MAGNESIUM: 8%

POTASSIUM: 400 mg

GOOD POINTS

Figs are a very good source of potassium and iron. Potassium is needed for proper muscle contractions (including those of the heart), for maintaining the correct fluid balance in the body, to help the transmission of nerve impulses, and for the release of energy from the carbohydrate and protein you eat. Iron is an essential part of hemoglobin in our blood and is needed to prevent anemia; approximately one-third of all young women get too little iron in their diets. Figs also contain vitamin B6 (which helps some women who suffer from PMS), calcium, magnesium, copper, and fiber (making them useful as laxative foods.)

BAD POINTS

Figs (especially dried ones) are very high in calories as well as simple sugars which can stick to the teeth and encourage tooth decay. These fruits are clearly not for anyone on a diet! Dried figs are often treated with SULFITES to preserve them. Some people are allergic to these substances and could develop symptoms such as rashes, watery eyes and breathing problems.

They also contain significant amounts of a substance called TYRAMINE, which can be very dangerous when consumed by someone who is taking monoamine oxidase inhibitors (MAOI's), a group of antidepressant medications.

FLOUNDER
(BAKED)

Serving Size: 3.5 ounces
Rating: ★★★

CALORIES: 237 mg
FAT: 8.2 grams
SODIUM: 237 mg
VITAMIN B3: 13%
IRON: 8%
IODINE: 10%
MAGNESIUM: 8%
PHOSPHORUS: 34%
POTASSIUM: 587 mg
PROTEIN: 67%

GOOD POINTS
Flounder is an excellent source of high quality protein, required for the growth and maintenance of all your body tissues. For a main course, it is also not especially high in calories. The fat it contains is mainly polyunsaturated and rich in the omega-3-fatty acids, which are believed to lower blood cholesterol levels. Flounder is also a good source of vitamin B3, phosphorus, potassium, magnesium, iron, and iodine. All health-conscious eaters should try to get fish into their diet at least three times a week.

BAD POINTS
Flounder is relatively high in calories (though certainly not terrible for a main course), fat and sodium. Fish is also sometimes implicated in ALLERGIC REACTIONS.

FRANKFURTER

Serving Size: 1
Rating: ★

CALORIES: 145
CHOLESTEROL: 22 mg
FAT: 13.2 grams
SODIUM: 461 mg
B COMPLEX VITAMINS: 6% for B3, 12% for B12
VITAMIN C: 18%
POTASSIUM: 71 mg
PROTEIN: 11%
ZINC: 6%

GOOD POINTS

The old ballpark favorite is a surprisingly good source of vitamin C, needed for healthy gums, teeth, bones, and muscles. Vitamin C may also help protect you from cancer and keep your immune system in good working order. In addition, franks contain vitamin B3, B12, potassium, zinc, and protein in significant amounts.

BAD POINTS

Hot dogs are high in calories, saturated fat, cholesterol, and sodium. If you're a heart-smart, health conscious eater, or a weight-watcher, you might want to bring a piece of fruit to the game instead!

Frankfurters are also high in nitrates, which may increase your risk of getting stomach cancer (although the vitamin C content should protect you to some extent).

FRENCH TOAST

Serving Size: 1 slice
Rating: ★★

CALORIES: 153
CHOLESTEROL: 17 mg
FAT: 6.7 grams
SODIUM: 257 mg
B COMPLEX VITAMINS: 8% for B1, 9% for B2, 5% for

B3, 5% for B12, 5% for pantothenic acid, and
5% for folic acid

CALCIUM: 7%

COMPLEX CARBOHYDRATE: 17.2 grams

IRON: 7%

PHOSPHORUS: 9%

POTASSIUM: 86 mg

PROTEIN: 13%

GOOD POINTS

French toast—not the best of breakfast choices but
certainly not the worst—contains good amounts of
the B vitamins (needed for getting energy from your
food, keeping your eyes and skin healthy, and for
many reactions in the brain), protein, calcium,
phosphorus, iron, and potassium.

BAD POINTS

It is very high in calories and contains significant
amounts of saturated fat and cholesterol. It is also
quite high in sodium. The bread used to make it
contains a substance called GLUTEN which can
cause an upset digestive system, anemia, weight loss,
bone pain, skin problems, and water retention in
people with a condition known as celiac disease.

FRUIT COCKTAIL

*Serving Size: ¹/₂ cup (canned in its own
juice)*
Rating: ★

CALORIES: 56

FAT: None

SIMPLE CARBOHYDRATE: 15 grams

VITAMIN A: 8%

VITAMIN C: 5%

POTASSIUM: 118 mg

GOOD POINTS

Fruit cocktail contains a small amount of vitamin A
(in the form of carotene) providing protection against
certain types of cancers, as well as keeping your skin,

hair, teeth, eyes, bones, glands and immune system in good working order. In addition, it is low in calories and has some vitamin C and potassium.

BAD POINTS

Fruit cocktail is high in simple sugars (which contribute to tooth decay) if it is canned in its own juice, but even worse if canned in syrup (which doubles both the sugar content and the calories).

GARLIC

Serving Size: 1 teaspoon (dried) or 1 clove
Rating: ★

CALORIES: 9
FAT: none

GOOD POINTS

Although raw garlic contains significant amounts of B complex vitamins, C, and potassium, iron, protein, and fiber, you will never eat enough of it to make a real impact on your body. Even a whole teaspoon doesn't have enough of anything to make a real health difference. Some research shows that consuming a level equivalent to 10 cloves a day could lower blood cholesterol levels.

BAD POINTS

Eating a lot of garlic can cause body and mouth odor due to the presence of a compound called diallyl sulfide in your perspiration and breath.

GOOSE

Serving Size: 3.5 ounces
Rating: ★★

CALORIES: 305

CHOLESTEROL: 91 mg

FAT: 21.9 grams

SODIUM: 70 mg

B COMPLEX VITAMINS: 5% for B1, 19% for B2, 21% for B3, and 19% for B6

COPPER: 13%

IRON: 16%

MAGNESIUM: 6%

PHOSPHORUS: 27%

POTASSIUM: 329 mg

PROTEIN: 56%

GOOD POINTS

Goose is an excellent source of good quality protein required for the growth and maintenance of all your body tissues, as well as well-absorbed iron (an essential part of hemoglobin in our blood, needed to prevent anemia). It is also a good place to find many B complex vitamins, potassium, phosphorus, magnesium, and copper.

BAD POINTS

Goose is relatively high in calories, saturated fat and cholesterol, making it a less than ideal choice for both weight and health watchers. Taking off the skin reduces the caloric content by one third but does little to change the cholesterol content. It also contains some sodium.

GRAPES

(SEEDLESS, GREEN)

Serving Size: 1 cup (10 grapes)
Rating: ★★

CALORIES: 58
FAT: 0.3 grams
SIMPLE CARBOHYDRATE: 15.8 grams
B COMPLEX VITAMINS: 6% for B1, 5% for B6
VITAMIN C: 6%
FIBER: .7 grams (from the skin)
POTASSIUM: 176 mg

GOOD POINTS

Grapes are low in calories and contain a good amount of potassium, along with some vitamin C, B1, B6 and fiber. Potassium is needed for proper muscle contractions (including those of the heart), for maintaining the correct fluid balance in the body, to help the transmission of nerve impulses, and for the release of energy from the carbohydrate and protein you eat. Instead of ice cream or cakes, try 10 frozen grapes as a healthy dessert treat!

BAD POINTS

Grapes are high in simple carbohydrate, which can cause tooth decay.

GRAPEFRUIT

Serving Size: 1/2 medium
Rating: ★★★

CALORIES: 39
FAT: 0.1 grams
SIMPLE CARBOHYDRATE: 9.9 grams
VITAMIN A (AS CAROTENE): 6% (red or pink fruit only)
VITAMIN C: 65 mg
FIBER: .2 grams (from flesh); .5 grams (from pith)
POTASSIUM: 175 mg

GOOD POINTS

Grapefruit is an excellent source of vitamin C, needed for healthy gums, teeth, bones, and muscles. (It may also help protect you from cancer and keep your immune system in good working order.) This excellent breakfast or lunch choice also contains a good amount of potassium. There is some fiber in the fleshy part and the pith; the pith contains the type of fiber known as pectin, which can lower blood cholesterol levels. While grapefruit is low in calories, it does not have a magic ability to "burn off fat," as some health faddist have proposed. The red (or pink) variety contains a good amount of vitamin A, as well, in the form of carotene.

BAD POINTS

The sweetness of grapefruit comes from simple carbohydrates, which can cause tooth decay. The peel contains oils that can cause SKIN IRRITATION in susceptible people.

GRAVY

Serving Size: ¹/₂ cup
Rating: Sorry, no stars

CALORIES: 9–164
SODIUM: 9–862 mg
FAT: 0.3 grams (au jus) to 8.5 grams (chicken)
POTASSIUM: 3–162 mg

GOOD POINTS

The composition of gravies is extremely variable, but some do contain significant amounts of potassium. However, none contain much else, and the negative aspects of this food can be so pronounced that it cannot be recommended as a health-giving selection.

BAD POINTS

Gravies can be extremely high in calories (as with thick brown ones) or extremely low (as with the clear au jus type). They can also be quite high in sodium (this time the au jus type is the culprit) or relatively low (as with the thick brown kind).

HADDOCK
(BROILED)

Serving Size: 3.5 ounces
Rating: ★★★★

CALORIES: 98

FAT: 6.6 grams

SODIUM: 71 mg

VITAMIN A: 6%

B COMPLEX VITAMINS: 10% for B3, 13% for B6, 17% for B12

VITAMIN C: 5%

CALORIES: 98

IODINE: 93%

POTASSIUM: 356 mg

PROTEIN: 44%

GOOD POINTS

This fish is an excellent source of high quality protein (required for the growth and maintenance of all your body tissues), and iodine (needed for the manufacture of thyroid hormone). It is very low in calories and contains significant amounts of potassium, vitamins A, B3, B6, B12, and C. Haddock is a low fat fish with omega-3 fatty acids, which tend to lower blood cholesterol levels. Health-conscious eaters should try to get fish like haddock into their diets at least three times a week.

BAD POINTS

Haddock contains a little fat and sodium. Fish is sometimes the cause of ALLERGIC SYMPTOMS such as stomach upset, hives, and swelling of the face, lips and eyes.

HALIBUT
(BROILED)

Serving Size: 3.5 ounces
Rating: ★★★

CALORIES: 131
FAT: 4 grams
SODIUM: 110 mg
B COMPLEX VITAMINS: 5% for B1, 6% for B2, 5.2% or B3, 9% for B6, and 17% for B12
IODINE: 10%
POTASSIUM: 340 mg
PROTEIN: 53%

GOOD POINTS
Halibut is an excellent source of good quality protein, required for the growth and maintenance of all your body tissues. It is also relatively low in calories and contains good quantities of potassium, vitamins B1, B2, B3, B6, B12, and iodine. It contains the omega-3 fatty acids, which can lower blood cholesterol. Health-conscious eaters should try to get fish like halibut into their diets at least three times a week.

BAD POINTS
Halibut contains some fat and sodium. Fish can be the cause of ALLERGIC SYMPTOMS such as stomach upset, hives, and swelling of the face, lips and eyes.

HAM

Serving Size: 1 slice (approx. 1.5 ounces)
Rating: ★★

CALORIES: 130
CHOLESTEROL: 50 mg
FAT: 4.7 grams
B COMPLEX VITAMINS: 23% for B1, 9% for B2, 12% for B3

IRON: 7%
PHOSPHORUS: 15%
POTASSIUM: 260 mg
PROTEIN: 44%

GOOD POINTS
Ham is a good source of high quality protein, required for the growth and maintenance of all your body tissues. It also contains impressive amounts of many B vitamins, as well as some potassium, phosphorus, and iron.

BAD POINTS
Ham contains about as much cholesterol as beef, but since its fat content is higher in polyunsaturates then saturates, it is slightly better. It is very high in calories; consider that 3 slices of ham is almost 400 calories, or about one-third of most women's daily calorie allowance!

HERRING
(PICKLED)

Serving Size: 3.5 ounces
Rating: ★

CALORIES: 223
CHOLESTEROL: 80 mg
FAT: 15.1 grams
SODIUM: 170 mg
IODINE: 10%
PROTEIN: 45%
POTASSIUM: 370 mg

GOOD POINTS
Herring is an excellent source of good quality protein, required for the growth and maintenance of all your body tissues. It also contains some iodine and potassium.

BAD POINTS
You may not have suspected it, but herring is pretty high in calories. It is also rich in fat and cholesterol,

although it does contain omega-3 fatty acids, which can lower blood cholesterol, and the fat is mainly monounsaturated and polyunsaturated. Herring also contains some sodium. Fish is sometimes the cause of ALLERGIC SYMPTOMS such as stomach upset, hives, and swelling of the face, lips and eyes.

HONEY

Serving Size: 1 tablespoon
Rating: Nope, no stars

CALORIES: 61
FAT: None
SIMPLE CARBOHYDRATE: 16.5 grams

GOOD POINTS
None, except for its lack of fat.

BAD POINTS
Many people are under the mistaken impression that honey is somehow better for you than white sugar. The fact is that it's high in calories, and composed of simple sugars with little else. On rare occasions, it contains botulinum spores that can develop in the intestines of infants and young children (but not adults) into the C. botulinum organism, causing a deadly form of FOOD POISONING. Honey collected in the wild—not commercially produced—can also cause FOOD ALLERGIES.

HORSERADISH

Serving Size: 1 tablespoon
Rating: ★

CALORIES: 7
FAT: none
POTASSIUM: 52 mg

GOOD POINTS

Horseradish is actually a good choice for flavoring and garnish. It is very low in calories and contains a little potassium.

BAD POINTS

None.

ICE CREAM
(DAIRY AND NON-DAIRY)

Serving Size: 1 scoop
Rating: ★

	Dairy	Non-Dairy
CALORIES:	83	83
CHOLESTEROL:	10 mg	5 mg
FAT:	3.3 grams	4.1 grams
SIMPLE CARBOHYDRATE:	12.4 grams	10.3 grams
VITAMIN B2:	5%	5%
CALCIUM:	7%	6%
PHOSPHORUS:	5%	4%
POTASSIUM:	90 mg	80 mg

GOOD POINTS

Ice cream is a good source of calcium, needed to build bones and teeth and to keep bones strong. It also contains potassium, phosphorus, and vitamin B2. In many respects, non-dairy and dairy ice cream are about the same.

BAD POINTS

Ice cream is high in calories and simple carbohydrate, and contains some fat. Dairy ice cream is only slightly worse, since its fat content is 70% saturated as opposed to 54% in the non-dairy variety. Dairy ice cream also contains a little more cholesterol—but not as much as you think!.

JAM

Serving Size: 1 tablespoon
Rating: Nope, no stars

CALORIES: 55
FAT: none
SIMPLE CARBOHYDRATE: 14.2 grams

GOOD POINTS
None, except that it has no fat.

BAD POINTS
Jam is nothing more than a source of simple sugars and calories; eating too much can lead to an expanding waistline and decaying teeth.

JELLY

Serving Size: 1 tablespoon
Rating: Nope, no stars

CALORIES: 55
FAT: none
SIMPLE CARBOHYDRATE: 14.1 grams

GOOD POINTS
None, except that it has no fat.

BAD POINTS
Jelly, like jam, can disturb both waistline and teeth; it's nothing more than a source of calories and simple sugars.

KALE

Serving Size: ³/₄ cup (cooked)
Rating: ★★★★

CALORIES: 28
FAT: 0.4 grams
VITAMIN A (AS CAROTENE): 148%
VITAMIN C: 103%
CALCIUM: 13%
IRON: 7%
FIBER: 1.1 grams
PHOSPHORUS: 5%
POTASSIUM: 221 mg
PROTEIN: 5%

GOOD POINTS

Kale is an excellent source of vitamins A and C, both of which give you protection against cancer. It is also low in calories and contains more calcium, ounce for ounce, than milk. If that wasn't enough, this extremely healthy vegetable selection has potassium, iron, and phosphorus, as well as a little fiber and protein.

BAD POINTS

All cruciferous (belonging to the cabbage family) vegetables contain GOITROGENS—substances that hamper the production of thyroid hormones by the thyroid gland. This can cause an enlargement of the gland (goiter) in an attempt by the body to compensate for the reduced hormone production by increasing the amount of tissue available. However, people with healthy thyroids would have to eat a very large amount of these vegetables before they would have any kind of problem. This is only of concern for those with sluggish thyroid glands. Goitrogens break down when the vegetable is heated, and so even if you have a thyroid problem, you can eat as much of the cooked vegetable as you want.

KETCHUP
(TOMATO)

Serving Size: 1 tablespoon
Rating: Sorry, no stars

CALORIES: 16
FAT: 0.1 gram
SODIUM: 156 mg
POTASSIUM: 54 mg

GOOD POINTS
Ketchup is low in calories and contains a significant amount of potassium but is not a great food selection mainly because of its sodium content.

BAD POINTS
It contains a large amount of sodium and so is off-limits for people with high blood pressure or water retention problems.

KIDNEY

Serving Size: 3.5 ounces (braised)
Rating: ★★★

CALORIES: 252
CHOLESTEROL: 387 mg
FAT: 12 grams
SODIUM: 253 mg
VITAMIN A: 23%
B COMPLEX VITAMINS: 45% for B1, 270% for B2, 54% for B3, 6% for B6 250% for B12, and 10% for pantothenic acid
VITAMIN C: 17%
IRON: 73%
PHOSPHORUS: 24%
POTASSIUM: 324 mg
PROTEIN: 73%

GOOD POINTS
This is an excellent source of B vitamins, in particular B2 and B12. It is also a wonderful source of good

quality protein and easily-absorbable iron. It contains significant amounts of potassium, phosphorus, and vitamins C and A. Despite this wonderful nutritional resume, kidney should be eaten in extreme moderation because of its health risks (see below).

BAD POINTS
Kidney is extremely high in cholesterol, containing more in one serving than the American Heart Association recommends for the entire day! It is also high in calories, saturated fat, and sodium, making it a bad food choice for salt, heart, and waistline watchers.

LAMB
Serving Size: 3.5 ounces (broiled, weighed with bone)
Rating: ★★

CALORIES: 244
CHOLESTEROL: 70 mg
FAT: 20.4 grams
SODIUM: 50 mg
B COMPLEX VITAMINS: 6% for B1, 9% for B2, 20% for B3, 12% for B6 and 33% for B12
COPPER: 6%
IRON: 7%
PHOSPHORUS: 13%
POTASSIUM: 210 mg
PROTEIN: 15.2 grams
ZINC: 15%

GOOD POINTS
Lamb is a very good source of high quality protein and B vitamins, and a good source of iron, phosphorus, copper, zinc, and potassium. However, the bad points are significant and so this food should be eaten with caution and moderation.

BAD POINTS
Lamb is higher in cholesterol and saturated fat than poultry, pork, and most cuts of beef. It is also high

in calories and contains some sodium. All in all, it's off the list for people watching their weight or their arteries.

LASAGNA

Serving Size: 8 ounces

Rating: ★★

CALORIES: 300
CHOLESTEROL: 30 mg
FAT: 14 grams
SODIUM: 806 mg
VITAMIN A: 27%
B COMPLEX VITAMINS: 28% for B1, 19% for B2, 21% for B3
VITAMIN C: 10%
CALCIUM: 35%
COMPLEX CARBOHYDRATE: 32 grams
IRON: 25%
PHOSPHORUS: 44%
POTASSIUM: 477 mg
PROTEIN: 42%

GOOD POINTS
This tasty and filling dish is a good source of protein, calcium and phosphorus, is rich in B vitamins, vitamin A and potassium, and contains some vitamin C. It is also full of complex carbohydrates, making it a good food choice for marathon runners.

BAD POINTS
Lasagna is very high in calories and sodium, and high in saturated fat and cholesterol. It contains quite a lot of cheese and so LACTOSE INTOLERANT people should be careful: pasta also contains GLUTEN, and so people with this food sensitivity should also eat with caution. Milk and dairy products are often implicated in FOOD ALLERGIES.

Leeks

Serving Size: 3–4 (cooked)
Rating: ★★

CALORIES: 24
FAT: 0.3 grams
VITAMIN B6: 8%
VITAMIN C: 25%
CALCIUM: 6%
FIBER: 3.9 grams
IRON: 11%
POTASSIUM: 280 mg

GOOD POINTS
This vegetable is a good source of vitamin C, low in calories, and contains significant quantities of potassium, calcium, iron, vitamin B6, and fiber. Leek soup is a delicious and interesting alternative for cold winter nights.

BAD POINTS
Since leeks are part of the onion family, they contain SULFUR COMPOUNDS that can make your breath smell.

Lemon

Serving Size: 1 medium
Rating: ★★

CALORIES: 17
FAT: 0.2 grams
VITAMIN C: 52%
POTASSIUM: 80 mg

GOOD POINTS
Lemon is an excellent source of vitamin C, needed for healthy gums, teeth, bones, and muscles. It also contains significant amounts of potassium, and is low in calories.

BAD POINTS

The peel of lemons contains an oil (LIMONENE) that causes a rash called CONTACT DERMATITIS in susceptible people.

LEMONADE

Serving Size: 8 fluid ounces
Rating: ★ if from frozen concentrate; none if from mix or canned

	mix	frozen concentrate	canned
CALORIES:	89	94	91
CARBOHYDRATE:	22 g	23.9 grams	22.7 grams
FAT:	none	none	none
SODIUM:	—	—	92 mg
VITAMIN C:	15%	25%	37%
CALCIUM:	—	8%	—
COPPER:	—	34%	—
PHOSPHORUS:	—	9%	—
POTASSIUM:	—	100 mg	—

GOOD POINTS

Lemonade varies tremendously in its nutrient content, depending on which form it comes in. Frozen concentrate is the best, since it is rich in vitamin C and contains a good amount of calcium, phosphorus, potassium, and copper. Lemonade from a mix or can is rich in vitamin C, but nothing else.

BAD POINTS

All three forms of lemonade are high in calories when you consider their limited nutritional value. They also contain a lot of simple carbohydrates which can be harmful for your teeth, and canned lemonade has significant amounts of sodium.

LETTUCE

Serving Size: 3.5 ounces
Rating: ★★

CALORIES: 12
FAT: none
VITAMIN A: 20%
B COMPLEX VITAMINS: 5% for B1, 5% for B2, and 9%
   for folic acid
VITAMIN C: 25%
CALCIUM: 5%
FIBER: 1.5 grams
IRON: 7%
POTASSIUM: 240 mg

GOOD POINTS

This traditional salad vegetable is a good source of
vitamin C and vitamin A as carotene (the darker the
leaf the greater the A content), both of which provide
protection against cancer. Lettuce also contains de-
cent amounts of the B vitamins, potassium, iron, and
calcium as well as a little fiber. It is extremely low in
calories, which is why many dieters fill up on salads.
Loose leaf lettuce has the highest calcium and iron
level and Romaine lettuce has the most vitamin A
and vitamin C.

BAD POINTS

Lettuce contains NITRATES, which are converted in
the body into NITRITES and NITROSAMINES—
potential carcinogens (cancer-causing agents).

LIME

Serving Size: 1 medium
Rating: ★★

CALORIES: 20
FAT: 0.1 grams
VITAMIN C: 33%
POTASSIUM: 68 mg

GOOD POINTS

Limes are a very good source of vitamin C, needed for healthy gums, teeth, bones, and muscles. They also contain some potassium, and are low in calories. They contain substances called FUROCOUMARINS which make the skin less sensitive to light and helping to avoid severe sunburn.

BAD POINTS

The peel contains an oil (LIMONENE) which can cause a rash called CONTACT DERMATITIS in suspectible people.

LIVER, BEEF

Serving Size: 3.5 ounces (stewed)
Rating: ★★★

CALORIES: 229

CHOLESTEROL: 240

FAT: 10.6 grams

SODIUM: 184 mg

VITAMIN A: 1068%

B COMPLEX VITAMINS: 17% for B1, 246% for B2, 83% for B3, 26% for B6, 1800% for B12, 73% for folic acid, and 57% for pantothenic acid

VITAMIN C: 45%

VITAMIN D: 11%

COPPER: 115%

IRON: 49%

MAGNESIUM: 5%

PHOSPHORUS: 48%

POTASSIUM: 380 mg

PROTEIN: 59%

ZINC: 29%

GOOD POINTS

Liver is the most concentrated form of nutrients in our diet. It is the best dietary source of vitamin A, B2, B12, folic acid, iron and copper. It is very high in the other B complex vitamins, vitamin C, protein, potassium, phosphorus, and zinc; and if all this wasn't enough, it also contains some magnesium and vitamin D.

BAD POINTS

Liver is very high in cholesterol, though this type is not quite as bad as chicken or calf liver. It is also moderately high in calories and contains a considerable amount of fat. In addition, it contains significant amounts of a substance called TYRAMINE, which can be very dangerous when consumed by someone who is taking monoamine oxidase inhibitors (MAOI's), a group of antidepressant medications.

LIVER, CALF

Serving Size: 3.5 ounces (pan-fried)
Rating: ★★★

CALORIES: 254
CHOLESTEROL: 384 mg
FAT: 13.2 gram
SODIUM: 118 mg
VITAMIN A: 654%
B COMPLEX VITAMINS: 14% for B1, 247% for B2, 83% for B3, 37% for B6, 1450% for B12, 80% for folic acid, and 88% for pantothenic acid
VITAMIN C: 62%
VITAMIN D: 3%
COPPER: 600%
IRON: 42%
MAGNESIUM: 7%
PHOSPHORUS: 54%
POTASSIUM: 453 mg
PROTEIN: 60%
ZINC: 41%

GOOD POINTS

Liver is the most concentrated form of nutrients in our diet. It is the best dietary source of vitamin A, B2, B12, folic acid, iron and copper. It is very high in the other B complex vitamins, vitamin C, protein, potassium, phosphorus, and zinc; and if all this wasn't enough, it also contains some magnesium and vitamin D.

BAD POINTS
Liver is very high in cholesterol, moderately high in calories, and contains a considerable amount of fat. In addition, it contains significant amounts of a substance called TYRAMINE, which can be very dangerous when consumed by someone who is taking monoamine oxidase inhibitors (MAOI's), a group of antidepressant medications.

LIVER, CHICKEN

Serving Size: 3.5 ounces (simmered)
Rating: ★★★

CALORIES: 157
CHOLESTEROL: 490 mg
FAT: 5.5 grams
SODIUM: 51 mg
VITAMIN A: 328%
B COMPLEX VITAMINS: 10% for B1, 10% for B2, 23% for B3, 29% for B6, 317% for B12, 193% for folic acid, and 54% for pantothenic acid
VITAMIN C: 27%
VITAMIN D: 2%
COPPER: 19%
IRON: 47%
MAGNESIUM: 5%
PHOSPHORUS: 31%
POTASSIUM: 140 mg
PROTEIN: 54%
ZINC: 29%

GOOD POINTS
Any kind of liver contains the best dietary source of vitamin A, B2, B12, folic acid, iron and copper. It is very high in the other B complex vitamins, vitamin C, protein, potassium, phosphorus, pantothenic acid, and zinc; and if all this wasn't enough, it also contains some magnesium and vitamin D.

Chicken liver is neither particularly high nor low in calories.

BAD POINTS
Chicken liver is extremely high in cholesterol—even more so than calf's liver. It also contains some fat and sodium, along with a considerable amount of a substance called TYRAMINE, which can be very dangerous when consumed by someone who is taking monoamine oxidase inhibitors (MAOI's), a group of antidepressant medications.

LOBSTER

Serving Size: ³/₄ lb. (broiled or boiled)
Rating: ★★★

CALORIES: 139
CHOLESTEROL: 150 mg
FAT: 4.5 grams
SODIUM: 396 mg
B COMPLEX VITAMINS: 7% for B1, 9% for B3, 19% for pantothenic acid
CALCIUM: 7%
COPPER: 100%
VITAMIN E: 9%
IODINE: 10%
IRON: 5%
MAGNESIUM: 10%
PHOSPHORUS: 33%
POTASSIUM: 307 mg
PROTEIN: 60%
ZINC: 13%

GOOD POINTS
The king of the seafood dishes is an excellent source of high quality protein, copper, and phosphorus, and contains good amounts of potassium, calcium, magnesium, iron, iodine, zinc, vitamins B1, B3, E and pantothenic acid. Lobster is a low-calorie choice too, provided you don't dip it into oil or butter.

BAD POINTS
Unfortunately, lobster is high in cholesterol, although it does not contain that much fat and the fat

it has is rich in omega-3 fatty acids (which may offer protection against heart disease). However, if you dip the lobster into butter you can greatly increase the amount of cholesterol and fat you're consuming and as much as triple the caloric content.

Lobster also contains quite a lot of sodium and has been linked to ALLERGIES in susceptible people.

MACADAMIA NUTS

Serving Size: 6 medium (roasted)
Rating: No stars

CALORIES: 109
FAT: 11.7 grams

GOOD POINTS
These exotic and tasty nuts contain less than 5% of the RDA of vitamin E, protein, the B vitamins and small amounts of fiber—in other words, not very much considering their drawbacks.

BAD POINTS
Macadamias are high in calories and fat (mainly polyunsaturated and monosaturated). Although these types of fat tend to lower blood cholesterol levels, eating any kind may raise your risk of getting breast, uterine, endometrial, ovarian, prostate, and colon cancer. Nuts are often implicated in FOOD ALLERGIES. If the nuts are salted, they are high in sodium.

MACARONI

Serving Size: ³/₅ cup
Rating: ★ (★★★ if enriched)

	Regular	Enriched
CALORIES:	117	117
FAT:	0.7 g	0.7 grams
VITAMIN B1:	—	20%
VITAMIN B2:	—	8%

VITAMIN B 3:	—	12%
COMPLEX CARBOHYDRATE:	25 grams	25 grams
IRON:	—	6%
PHOSPHORUS:	5%	5%
POTASSIUM:	67 mg	67 mg
PROTEIN:	7%	7%

GOOD POINTS

This is a good food to fill up on, since it is high in complex carbohydrates and has negligible amounts of fat. It also contains a little protein, potassium, and phosphorus, and some products have added B vitamins and iron.

BAD POINTS

Macaroni contains a substance called GLUTEN which can cause an upset digestive system, anemia, weight loss, bone pain, skin problems, and water retention in people with a condition known as celiac disease.

MACKEREL

Serving Size: 1 fillet (broiled)
Rating: ★★★

CALORIES: 300
CHOLESTEROL: 104 mg
FAT: 20.5 grams
SODIUM: 169 mg
VITAMIN A: 14%
B COMPLEX VITAMINS: 13% for B1, 21% for B2, 49% for B3, 50% for B6, 217% for B12, 13% for pantothenic acid
COPPER: 12%
VITAMIN D: 200%
IODINE: 10%
IRON: 9%
MAGNESIUM: 10%
PHOSPHORUS: 36%
POTASSIUM: 485 mg
PROTEIN: 63%
ZINC: 5%

GOOD POINTS

This fish is extremely rich in protein, B vitamins, and vitamin D. It contains good amounts of iodine, iron, vitamin A, magnesium, copper, zinc, phosphorus, potassium, and iodine. This is the fish that has the most omega-3 fatty acids, which seem to reduce blood cholesterol levels.

BAD POINTS

Mackerel is high in calories, fat and cholesterol, and contains some sodium. Fish is sometimes the cause of ALLERGIC SYMPTOMS such as stomach upset, hives, and swelling of the face, lips and eyes.

MARGARINE

Serving Size: 1 teaspoon
Rating: Nope, no stars

CALORIES: 34
FAT: 3.8 grams
SODIUM: 51 MG

GOOD POINTS
None.

BAD POINTS

Margarine really does not contribute anything of value in the way of essential nutrients. It contains less than the RDA for vitamin A and E in a single serving, but a moderate amount of calories. The softer the margarine, the safer it is for you because the polyunsaturated and monounsaturated fat content is higher. When it is HYDROGENATED or HARDENED, some of the fat is changed to an unnatural form that may be harmful (some experts believe it could contribute to your risk for arteriosclerosis). Therefore, you should always look for the margarine with the lowest percent of hydrogenation. Salt-free margarine has less than 2 mg of sodium, but the regular kind contains significant amounts. In spite of all this, margarine should be used in preference to butter.

Matzo

Serving Size: 1
Rating: ★

CALORIES: 117
FAT: 0.9 grams
COMPLEX CARBOHYDRATE: 25.4 grams
FIBER: 1.5 grams
POTASSIUM: 50 mg
PROTEIN: 5%

GOOD POINTS

Matzo contains a significant amount of fiber (for the prevention of constipation and other related gastrointestinal disorders) along with some protein and potassium. Other than that, it is mainly carbohydrate in the form of starch.

BAD POINTS

Matzo is high in calories. It also contains a substance called GLUTEN which can cause an upset digestive system, anemia, weight loss, bone pain, skin problems, and water retention in people with a condition known as celiac disease.

Marmalade

Serving Size: 1 tablespoon
Rating: No stars

CALORIES: 56
FAT: none
SIMPLE CARBOHYDRATE: 14 grams

GOOD POINTS

None, except for its low fat content.

BAD POINTS

It contains 56 calories of pure sugar (which can be bad for your teeth), without traces of any essential nutrient.

MAYONNAISE

Serving Size: 1 tablespoon
Rating: Sorry, no stars

CALORIES: 99
FAT: 11 grams
SODIUM: 78 mg

GOOD POINTS
None.

BAD POINTS
Try lemon or vinegar on your tuna and salads, or go for low-calorie mayonnaise (which contains only 19 calories with very little fat and sodium). The regular type is high in calories and fat, and although the fat is mainly polyunsaturated (because mayonnaise is made from vegetable oils) eating too much of any type can increase your risk of getting cancer. Regular mayonnaise also contains significant amounts of sodium.

MELON, CANTALOUPE

Serving Size: 1 cup (pieces)
Rating: ★★★★

CALORIES: 57
FAT: 0.4
SIMPLE CARBOHYDRATES: 13 grams
VITAMIN A: 109%
B COMPLEX VITAMINS: 9% for B6, 7% for folic acid
VITAMIN C: 112%
POTASSIUM: 474 mg

GOOD POINTS
Cantaloupe contains over 100% of the USRDA for both vitamins A (as carotene) and C—the "anticancer" nutrients—and has significant amounts of B6, folic acid, and potassium. It makes the perfect appetizer and/or dessert. When the season is right,

try to get as much of this sweet-tasting and refreshing four-star food into your daily diet as you can.

BAD POINTS
Cantaloupe contains a significant amount of simple carbohydrate, which can cause tooth decay.

MELON, HONEYDEW
Serving Size: ¼ small (raw)
Rating:★★★★

CALORIES: 21
FAT: none
VITAMIN C: 42%
FIBER: 0.9 grams
FOLIC ACID: 8%
POTASSIUM: 220 mg

GOOD POINTS
This type of melon is an excellent source of vitamin C (important for healthy teeth, gums, blood vessels, bones and as protection against disease; it aids in iron absorption, and may help protect you against cancer). Honeydew also contains good amounts of potassium and folic acid, and is very low in calories. For your health and your weight, cut up pieces of melon for the perfect snack.

BAD POINTS
None.

MELON, WATERMELON
Serving Size: 1 cup
Rating: ★★

CALORIES: 50
FAT: 0.7 grams
SIMPLE CARBOHYDRATE: 11.5 grams
B COMPLEX VITAMINS: 9% for B1, 12% for B6

FIBER: 0.5 grams; much of it is in the form of
pectin, which lowers blood cholesterol
POTASSIUM: 186 mg

GOOD POINTS
This refreshing melon is a very good source of
vitamin C, needed for healthy gums, teeth, bones,
and muscles. It also contains good amounts of
vitamin B6, potassium, B1 and fiber, and is low in
calories.

BAD POINTS
It's high in simple carbohydrates, which can contribute to tooth decay.

MILK
Serving Size: 1 cup
Rating: ★★★ (if whole or 2%);
★★★★ (if skim or 1%)

	Skim	1% Fat	2% Fat	Whole
CALORIES:	86	102	121	150
CHOLESTEROL:	4 mg	10 mg	18 mg	33 mg
FAT:	2.6 grams	4.7 grams	6.4 grams	8.2 mg
SIMPLE CARBOHYDRATE (Mainly lactose):	11.9 grams	11.7 grams	11.7 grams	11.4 grams
SODIUM:	126 mg	123 mg	122 mg	120 mg
VITAMIN A:	15%	15%	15%	10–15%
VITAMIN B1:	6%	7%	7%	6%
VITAMIN B2:	20%	24%	24%	24%
VITAMIN B6:	5%	5%	5%	5%
VITAMIN B12:	16%	15%	15%	15%
PANTOTHENIC ACID:	8%	8%	8%	8%
CALCIUM:	30%	30%	30%	29%
VITAMIN D:	25%	25%	25%	25%
IODINE:	60%	60%	60%	60%
IRON:	6%	7%	7%	7%
MAGNESIUM:	7%	9%	8%	8%
PHOSPHORUS:	25%	24%	23%	23%
POTASSIUM:	406 mg	381 mg	377 mg	370 mg
PROTEIN:	19%	18%	18%	18%
ZINC:	7%	6%	6%	6%

GOOD POINTS

Milk is rich in many different nutrients. It is the best dietary source of calcium, needed to build bones and teeth and keep bones strong. (Your body absorbs calcium from milk and milk products better than from any other food source.) Milk also contains good amounts of iodine and vitamins A, B2, B12, and D, along with other B vitamins, potassium, phosphorus, protein, magnesium, iron and zinc. People now commonly get very different kinds of milk, many of which minimize the bad points mentioned below.

BAD POINTS

Milk can be high in calories—the higher the fat content, the higher the caloric value (whole milk has double the calories of skim milk). Whole milk also has significant amounts of fat and cholesterol. All types contain quite a bit of sodium.

Some people don't have an enzyme called lactase in their bodies, which is needed to break down milk sugar (lactose). As a result, when they eat dairy products, the lactose passes through the digestive system where it is broken down by bacteria instead, causing flatulence, bloating, and diarrhea. Allergies to the protein in milk, causing symptoms similar to those of lactose intolerance, also affect many people.

MOLASSES
(BLACKSTRAP)

Serving Size: 1 tablespoon
Rating: ★

CALORIES: 43
FAT: none
SIMPLE CARBOHYDRATE: 11 grams
CALCIUM: 12%
IRON: 13%

GOOD POINTS

Blackstrap molasses is a good choice for a sweetener since it contains both calcium (needed to build bones and teeth and to keep bones strong), and iron (an essential part of hemoglobin in our blood and needed to prevent anemia; approximately one-third of all young women get too little iron in their diets). Other types of molasses don't have as much of these nutrients.

BAD POINTS
Molasses is high in simple sugars (bad for your teeth) and calories.

MUFFIN

Serving Size: 1 whole
Rating: ★★ (if English or Bran) (if corn) ★

	English	Bran	Corn
CALORIES:	135	168	195
FAT:	1.1 grams	7.5 grams	6.3 grams
SODIUM:	364 mg	248 mg	465 mg
VITAMIN A:	—	6%	—
VITAMIN B1:	17%	10%	7%
VITAMIN B2:	11%	9%	7%
VITAMIN B3:	11%	10%	5%
VITAMIN B6:	—	8%	—
FOLIC ACID:	—	6%	—
CALCIUM:	9%	8%	15%
COPPER:	9%	7%	—
COMPLEX CARBOHYDRATE:	26.2grams	24 grams	30 grams
FIBER:	0.3 grams	0.5 grams	0.1 grams
IRON:	9%	11%	5%
MAGNESIUM:	—	13%	—
PHOSPHORUS:	6%	17%	23%
POTASSIUM:	319 mg	145 mg	66 mg
PROTEIN:	7%	7%	6%
ZINC:	—	11%	—

GOOD POINTS
Muffins contain significant amounts of the B vitamins, calcium, phosphorus, iron, copper, potassium, protein, zinc, fiber, and magnesium, but these

numbers vary considerably depending on which kind you select.

BAD POINTS
The fat content and caloric value of muffins vary tremendously among different types, with bran muffins and corn muffins being six or seven times higher in fat than English muffins. All types have a high sodium content.

With both bran and English muffins there is a danger of sensitivity to a substance called GLUTEN which can cause an upset digestive system, anemia, weight loss, bone pain, skin problems, and water retention in people with a condition known as celiac disease. Many people are ALLERGIC to corn.

MUSHROOM
Serving Size: 10 small (raw)
Rating: ★★★

CALORIES: 13
FAT: 0.6 grams
B COMPLEX VITAMINS: 7% for B1, 24% for B2, 20% for B3, 5% for B6, 6% for folic acid, and 20% for pantothenic acid
VITAMIN C: 5%
COPPER: 32%
FIBER: 2.5 grams
IRON: 5%
PHOSPHORUS: 14%
POTASSIUM: 470 mg

GOOD POINTS
Mushrooms are very low in calories and packed with many good nutrients. They are high in copper, B vitamins, potassium, phosphorus, and fiber. They also contain iron and vitamin C. However, all these benefits belong to raw mushrooms only: if you cook them they are nowhere near as healthy for you and if cooked in oil can be extremely high in calories.

BAD POINTS
If you harvest your own mushrooms, be careful, for as many as 100 out of the 1000 varieties are POISON-

OUS. Symptoms may appear from a few minutes to three days after you eat them, and can vary from salivation, cramps, diarrhea, vomiting, sweating, dizziness, and confusion, to convulsions, coma, and even death.

MUSSELS

Serving Size: 3.5 grams (boiled)
Rating: ★★

CALORIES: 87
CHOLESTEROL: 100 mg
FAT: 2.0 grams
CALCIUM: 20%
COPPER: 24%
IODINE: 10%
IRON: 43%
MAGNESIUM: 6%
PHOSPHORUS: 33%
POTASSIUM: 92 mg
PROTEIN: 38%
ZINC: 14%

GOOD POINTS
Mussels are low in fat, and a wonderful source of well-absorbed iron, protein, calcium, phosphorus, and copper. They also contain iodine, potassium, magnesium, and zinc. (If you weigh them with their shells, you will get approximately one-third of the amount of each nutrient listed for every 3.5 ounces.)

BAD POINTS
Mussels are very high in cholesterol, and contain quite a bit of sodium. Shellfish have also been implicated in ALLERGIES. They can be the cause of HEPATITIS and RED TIDE POISONING.

MUSTARD

Serving Size: 1 tablespoon
Rating: No stars

CALORIES: 5
FAT: 0.3 grams
SODIUM: 65 mg

GOOD POINTS
About the only good thing you can say about mustard is that it's extremely low in calories.

BAD POINTS
Mustard is very high in sodium, making it the wrong condiment for people for salt-restricted diets.

NECTARINE

Serving Size: 1 medium
Rating: ★★

CALORIES: 67
FAT: 0.6 grams
SIMPLE CARBOHYDRATES: 16.0 grams
VITAMIN A: 20%
VITAMIN B3: 7%
FIBER: 0.5 grams; some of it is in the form of pectin, which lowers blood cholesterol (the less ripe the tangerine, the greater the amount of pectin)
POTASSIUM: 288 mg

GOOD POINTS
This fruit is a very good source of vitamin A in the form of carotene, which offers some protection against cancer and is good for your skin, hair, and eyes. It also contains some vitamin C, B3, quite a lot of potassium, and a little fiber. It is neither especially high nor low in calories.

BAD POINTS
Nectarines are high in simple sugars, which can contribute to tooth decay.

NOODLES

(ENRICHED)

Serving Size: ³/₅ cup (cooked)
Rating: ★★

CALORIES: 120

FAT: 1.5 grams

B COMPLEX VITAMINS: 20% for B1, 8% for B2, and 11% for B3

COMPLEX CARBOHYDRATE: 20.1 grams

IRON: 8%

MAGNESIUM: 5%

PHOSPHORUS: 6%

POTASSIUM: 53mg

PROTEIN: 6%

GOOD POINTS

Noodles are a good source of several of the B vitamins (1, 2 & 3), needed for getting energy from your food, keeping your eyes and skin healthy, and for many reactions in the brain; along with iron, an essential part of hemoglobin in our blood and needed to prevent anemia. They also contain significant amounts of protein, phosphorus, potassium, and magnesium.

BAD POINTS

Noodles are high in calories and contain a substance called GLUTEN which can cause an upset digestive system, anemia, weight loss, bone pain, skin problems, and water retention in people with a condition known as celiac disease.

OILS

Serving Size: 1 tablespoon
Rating: No stars

CALORIES: 120

FAT: 13.6 grams

GOOD POINTS

Vegetable oils (except for coconut oil) are preferable to butter, margarine, and other hard fats as they have a lower level of saturated fat and a higher level of monounsaturated and polyunsaturated fat. Saturated fat raises blood cholesterol levels while the latter two types lower it; however, eating any sort of fat seems to increase your risk of getting breast, uterine, endometrial, ovarian, prostate, and colon cancer. The table below lists the most predominant types of fat found in the various cooking oils.

Oil	Monounsaturated	Polyunsaturated	Saturated
Coconut			X
Corn		X	
Cottonseed		X	
Olive	X		
Palm	X		
Peanut	X	X	
Safflower		X	
Sesame		X	
Soybean		X	
Sunflower		X	

BAD POINTS

Oils are pure fat and so increase your risk of getting certain types of cancer (see above). They are also high in calories.

OKRA

Serving Size: 8–9 pods
Rating: ★★★★

CALORIES: 29
FAT: none
VITAMIN A: 10%
B COMPLEX VITAMINS: 9% for B1, 11% for B2, 5% for B3, and 20% for folic acid
VITAMIN C: 33%
CALCIUM: 9%
COMPLEX CARBOHYDRATE: 6 grams
COPPER: 10%

FIBER: 2 grams; most of it is in the form of pectin, which lowers blood cholesterol

IRON: 6%

MAGNESIUM: 15%

PHOSPHORUS: 6%

POTASSIUM: 174 mg

GOOD POINTS

This vegetable is a real nutrient bonanza! It's an excellent source of vitamin C (needed for healthy gums, teeth, bones, and muscles) and a very good source of folic acid, magnesium, potassium, copper, vitamins A and B2. It also contains significant amounts of fiber, vitamin B1 and B3, calcium, iron, and phosphorus, as well as being low in calories. Okra is a good choice for thickening soups and stews.

BAD POINTS

None.

OLIVES

*Serving Size: 2 large black
or 3 medium green
or 3 medium Greek
Rating: Sorry, no stars*

	Black	Green	Greek
CALORIES:	37	23	67
FAT:	4 grams	2.4 grams	7.1 grams
SODIUM:	150 mg	418 mg	658 mg
FIBER	.3 grams	.3 grams	.8 grams

GOOD POINTS

Olives only contain a little fiber.

BAD POINTS

Olives are high in sodium, especially the Greek variety which have four times as much as the black kind. Greek olives are also very high in calories. All types contain monounsaturated fat, which helps reduce your cholesterol level, but like other fats increases your cancer risk.

ONIONS

Serving Size: 1 medium (raw)
Rating: ★★

CALORIES: 38
FAT: 0.4 grams
VITAMIN B6: 5%
VITAMIN C: 17%
FIBER: 1.3 grams
POTASSIUM: 157 mg

GOOD POINTS
Onions are a very good source of vitamin C (needed for healthy gums, teeth, bones, and muscles), and a good source of potassium and fiber. They also contain some vitamin B6 and are extremely low in calories. If you eat the green tips of spring onions, you will get a lot of vitamin A in the form of carotene (an anti-cancer nutrient).

BAD POINTS
Onions contain SULFUR COMPOUNDS that can make your breath smell; the fresher the onion the higher the content of these substances. Cooking breaks down these compounds and reduces the problem.

ORANGES

Serving Size: 1 medium
Rating: ★★★

CALORIES: 59
FAT: none
SIMPLE CARBOHYDRATE: 14.4 grams
VITAMIN A: 6%
B COMPLEX VITAMINS: 7% for B1, 12% for folic acid

VITAMIN C: 100%

CALCIUM: 5%

COPPER: 5%

FIBER: 0.6 grams; some of it is in the form of pectin, which lowers blood cholesterol

POTASSIUM: 217 mg

GOOD POINTS

Oranges are of course an excellent source of vitamin C (needed for healthy gums, teeth, bones, and muscles) provided you don't peel them too much, since most of the C content is in the white layer just under the skin. They also contain good amounts of folic acid and potassium, as well as some vitamin A, vitamin B1, potassium, calcium, copper, and fiber.

BAD POINTS

Oranges contain simple sugars that can cause tooth decay. They also contain a natural substance that may cause a rash called CONTACT DERMATITIS in susceptible people.

ORANGE JUICE

Serving Size: 8 fluid ounces (fresh)
Rating: ★★★

CALORIES: 111

FAT: 0.4 grams

SIMPLE CARBOHYDRATE: 25.8 grams

VITAMIN A: 10%

B COMPLEX VITAMINS: 15% for B1, 5% for B6, 28% for folic acid, and 5% for pantothenic acid

VITAMIN C: 200%

COPPER: 5%

MAGNESIUM: 7%

POTASSIUM: 496 mg

GOOD POINTS

All types of orange juice are excellent sources of vitamin C but fresh has the edge over the kind made from concentrate or canned. All types are also very good sources of potassium (making it a natural diuretic), folic acid, and vitamin B1, as well as containing significant amounts of vitamin A (fresh and canned have twice as much as frozen concentrate). Orange juice also has magnesium, pantothenic acid, copper, B6, and the canned type contains a little iron (6% of the RDA).

BAD POINTS
Orange juice is pretty high in calories and simple sugars (which can cause tooth decay). It's a good idea to drink orange juice through a straw to limit contact with teeth. For the same reason, a teething baby should never be left for a long time with a bottle containing orange juice.

OYSTERS
Serving Size: 5–8 medium (raw)
Rating: ★★

CALORIES: 66
CHOLESTEROL: 20 mg
FAT: 2.1 grams
SODIUM: 73 mg
VITAMIN A: 6%
B COMPLEX VITAMINS: 9% for B1, 11% for B2, 13% for B3
CALCIUM: 9%
IODINE: 93%
IRON: 31%
MAGNESIUM: 8%
PHOSPHORUS: 14%
POTASSIUM: 121 mg
PROTEIN: 19%
ZINC: 36%

GOOD POINTS
Oysters do not seem to affect sexual potency (contrary to popular myth) but they are low in calories, an excellent source of iodine, zinc, iron, and a good source of protein, vitamin B3, and phosphorus. They also contain significant amounts of vitamins A, B1, and B2, potassium, magnesium, and calcium.

BAD POINTS

They are very high in cholesterol and contain a little sodium. Also, shellfish have been implicated in ALLERGIES and can be the cause of HEPATITIS and RED TIDE POISONING.

PANCAKES
(PLAIN)

Serving Size: 1 medium
Rating: ★

CALORIES: 104
FAT: 3.2 grams
SODIUM: 191 mg
VITAMIN B2: 6%
CALCIUM: 5%
COMPLEX CARBOHYDRATE: 15.3 grams
PHOSPHORUS: 6%
POTASSIUM: 53 mg
PROTEIN: 5%

GOOD POINTS

Pancakes have some protein, vitamin B2, calcium, phosphorus, and potassium, but are not a particularly good source of anything when you consider how many calories they contain!

BAD POINTS

This traditional breakfast food is unfortunately high in calories, sodium, and contains some saturated fat. Since pancakes also contain milk, they can cause symptoms like flatulence, bloating, and diarrhea in people who are LACTOSE INTOLERANT. ALLERGIES to the protein in milk, causing symptoms similar to those of lactose intolerance, affect many people. Pancakes also contain a substance called GLUTEN which can cause an upset digestive system, anemia, weight loss, bone pain, skin problems, and water retention in people with a condition known as celiac disease.

PANCAKES
(BUCKWHEAT)

Serving Size: 1 medium
Rating: ★

CALORIES: 90
FAT: 3.2 grams
SODIUM: 209 mg
VITAMIN B2: .12 mg
CALCIUM: 5%
COMPLEX CARBOHYDRATE: 15.3 grams
PHOSPHORUS: 15%
POTASSIUM: 110 mg
PROTEIN: 5%

GOOD POINTS

Pancakes have some protein, vitamin B2, calcium, phosphorus, and potassium, but are not a particularly good source of anything when you consider how many calories they contain!

BAD POINTS

This traditional breakfast food is unfortunately high in calories, sodium, and contains some saturated fat. Since pancakes also contain milk, they can cause symptoms like flatulence, bloating, and diarrhea in people who are LACTOSE INTOLERANT. ALLERGIES to the protein in milk, causing symptoms similar to those of lactose intolerance, affect many people. Pancakes also contain a substance called GLUTEN which can cause an upset digestive system, anemia, weight loss, bone pain, skin problems, and water retention in people with a condition known as celiac disease.

PAPAYA

Serving Size: ¹/₂ medium
Rating: ★★★

CALORIES: 58

FAT: 0.2 grams

SIMPLE CARBOHYDRATE: 15 grams

VITAMIN A: 61%

VITAMIN C: 157%

FIBER: 1.2 grams; some of it is in the form of pectin, which lowers blood cholesterol

GOOD POINTS

This exotic, delicious fruit is low in calories, an excellent source of vitamins A (as carotene) and C—both of which can protect you against cancer—and a good source of potassium. It also contains some fiber.

BAD POINTS

Papayas are high in simple sugars which can cause tooth decay. Unripe papayas contain PAPAIN, an enzyme that breaks down protein. This can cause a rash called DERMATITIS, but in this case it is not just an allergic reaction but something that can be a problem for anyone.

PARSLEY

Serving Size: 1 tablespoon
Rating: ★★★

CALORIES: 4

FAT: 0.1 gram

VITAMIN A: 17%

VITAMIN C: 28%

POTASSIUM: 73 mg

GOOD POINTS

Freshly chopped parsley, as a garnish or in salads, is a very good source of vitamin A (as carotene) and

C—both of which can protect you against cancer—and contains some potassium. However, dried parsley has fewer of these nutrients.

BAD POINTS
None.

PATÉ

Serving Size: 1 ounce
Rating: ★

CALORIES: 90
CHOLESTEROL: 43 mg
FAT: 7.9 grams
SODIUM: 198 mg
VITAMIN A: 19%
B COMPLEX VITAMINS: 10% for B2, 15% for B12
COPPER: 6%
IRON: 9%
PHOSPHORUS: 6%
PROTEIN: 9%

GOOD POINTS
Paté is a very good source of vitamins A and B12; it also contains significant amounts of protein and B2, as well as phosphorus, iron and copper. The new vegetable-based patés have fewer of the serious drawbacks listed below, but depending on what is used, can contain less of these nutrients.

BAD POINTS
It is quite high in calories, saturated fat, and cholesterol, even though many people eat it because they believe it is somehow healthier and less caloric than most other foods. As a general rule, you can remember that the more expensive the paté, the higher its fat and cholesterol content. It is also pretty rich in sodium, and so off the menu for salt-watchers.

PEAS

	Fresh	Canned	Frozen
CALORIES:	52	41	47
FAT:	0.2 grams	0.2 grams	0.1 grams
VITAMIN A			
(AS CAROTENE):	10%	8%	14%
VITAMIN B1:	19%	7%	20%
VITAMIN B2:	6%	5%	6%
VITAMIN B3:	12%	5%	11%
FOLIC ACID:	20%	7%	22%
VITAMIN C:	33%	18%	33%
COMPLEX			
CARBOHYDRATE:	7.7 grams	7 grams	4 grams
COPPER:	8%	6%	6%
FIBER:	2.0 grams	1.4 grams	2.0 grams
IRON:	10%	6%	9%
MAGNESIUM:	5%	5%	5%
PHOSPHORUS:	10%	6%	9%
POTASSIUM:	196 mg	112 mg	149 mg
PROTEIN:	8%	7%	8%
ZINC:	5%	5%	5%

GOOD POINTS
Peas are low in calories, a very good source of vitamin
C as well as A (as carotene)—both anti-cancer
nutrients—and contain significant amounts of B
vitamins, potassium, iron, phosphorus, copper, zinc,
protein, magnesium, and fiber.

BAD POINTS
Canned peas may have a hefty 230 mg of SODIUM
added to them.

Peach

Serving Size: 1 medium (raw)
Rating: ★

CALORIES: 37
FAT: 0.1 gram
VITAMIN A: 9%
VITAMIN C: 10%
FIBER: 0.6 grams in the form of pectin, which can lower blood cholesterol
POTASSIUM: 171 mg

GOOD POINTS

Peaches contain a good amount of vitamin A as carotene and vitamin C—both nutrients can offer protection against cancer—as well as potassium. They are also low in calories and contain some pectin-type fiber (the cholesterol-lowering kind); however, the riper the peach, the less the fiber content since this fiber is converted into sugar as the fruit ripens.

BAD POINTS

Peaches contain GOITROGENS—substances that hamper the production of thyroid hormones by the thyroid gland. This can cause an enlargement of the gland (goiter) in an attempt by the body to compensate for the reduced hormone production by increasing the amount of tissue available. However, people with healthy thyroids would have to eat a very large amount of this fruit before they would have any kind of problem. This is only of concern for those with sluggish thyroid glands.

Dried peaches are often treated with SULFITES to preserve them (prevent them from darkening in color). Some people are allergic to these substances, and could develop symptoms such as rashes, watery eyes, and breathing problems.

Peach pits contain AMYGDALIN, a naturally-occurring substance that breaks down into hydrogen cyanide. While accidentally swallowing a peach pit is not a problem, taking in a greater amount could be hazardous and even a small amount could be lethal in a very small child.

PEANUTS

Serving Size: 1 ounce
Rating: ★★

	Fresh	Roasted
CALORIES:	157	170
FAT:	13.2 grams	14 grams
SODIUM:	—	138 mg (if added)
VITAMIN B1:	16%	5%
VITAMIN B3:	27%	27%
VITAMIN B6:	8%	6%
FOLIC ACID:	9%	—
COPPER:	11%	11%
VITAMIN E:	41%	41%
FIBER:	0.5 grams	0.5 grams
IRON:	6%	6%
MAGNESIUM:	11%	11%
PHOSPHORUS:	13%	13%
POTASSIUM:	210 mg	210 mg
PROTEIN:	12%	12%
ZINC:	6%	6%

GOOD POINTS

Peanuts are an excellent source of vitamin E, which has an important role to play in protecting our cell membranes from wear and tear, and helping to prevent the formation of free radicals (substances believed to be a cause of cancer). E may also facilitate the healing of wounds and burns when applied topically. Peanuts contain several B vitamins, magnesium, potassium, phosphorus, and copper, as well as good amounts of protein, iron, zinc and a little fiber (a lot if you eat the skins). Roasting tends to reduce the levels of some of these nutrients.

BAD POINTS

Peanuts are high in calories and fat, mainly polyunsaturated and monounsaturated. Although these types tend to lower blood cholesterol levels, eating any sort of fat seems to raise your risk of getting breast, uterine, endometrial, ovarian, prostrate, and colon cancer. If peanuts are roasted with salt, they also contain a considerable amount of sodium. They are often the cause of ALLERGIC REACTIONS in susceptible people.

PEAR

Serving Size: 1 medium (raw)
Rating: ★

CALORIES: 98
FAT: 0.7 grams
SIMPLE CARBOHYDRATE: 25.1 grams
VITAMIN C: 12%
COPPER: 9%
FIBER: 2.3 grams; some of it is in the form of pectin, which lowers blood cholesterol
POTASSIUM: 208 mg

GOOD POINTS
Pears contain good amounts of potassium, copper, vitamin C, and fiber. Most of the vitamin C and a great deal of the fiber are in the skin.

BAD POINTS
Pears have a lot of simple sugars, which makes them a fairly high calorie fruit. They contain GOITROGENS—substances that hamper the production of thyroid hormones by the thyroid gland. This can cause an enlargement of the gland (goiter) in an attempt by the body to compensate for the reduced hormone production by increasing the amount of tissue available. However, people with healthy thyroids would have to eat a very large amount of pears before they would have any kind of problem. This is only of concern for those with sluggish thyroid glands.

The pits of pears contain AMYGDALIN, a naturally-occuring substance that breaks down into hydrogen cyanide. While accidentally swallowing a pear seed is not a problem, taking in a large number could be hazardous and even a few seeds could be lethal in a very small child.

Dried pears are often sprayed with SULFITES to preserve them. Some people are allergic to these substances, and could develop symptoms such as rashes, watery eyes, and breathing problems.

PECAN

Serving Size: 12 halves
Rating: ★

CALORIES: 104
FAT: 11 grams
VITAMIN B1: 7%
PHOSPHORUS: 5%
POTASSIUM: 90 mg

GOOD POINTS
Pecans contain some potassium, vitamin B1, and phosphorus.

BAD POINTS
Pecans are high in fat and calories. Although the fat is monosaturated and polyunsaturated and tends to reduce blood cholesterol levels it can still be a problem; any type of fat seems to raise your risk of getting breast, uterine, endometrial, ovarian, prostate, and colon cancer. If the nuts are salted they can also be high in sodium. Nuts are often implicated in ALLERGIC REACTIONS.

PEPPER

Serving Size: 1 cup (sliced)
Rating: ★★★

	Green	Red	Chili
CALORIES:	18	25	49
FAT:	0.1 grams	0.1 grams	0.1 grams
VITAMIN A:	7%	71%	30%
VITAMIN C:	170%	272%	278%
POTASSIUM:	170 mg	170 mg	170 mg

GOOD POINTS

Sweet peppers or bell peppers are green when immature and red when mature. Both types are low in calories, excellent sources of vitamin C and very good sources of potassium. As peppers mature, their content of both vitamin C and A increases dramatically; both vitamins may provide some protection against cancer. Chili peppers are also excellent source of all these nutrients.

BAD POINTS

You should use gloves when cutting up hot peppers: They contain large amounts of chemicals called CAPSAICIN, NORDIHYDROCAPSAICIN, and DIHYDROCAPSAICIN, which will burn your hands. These chemicals cannot be washed off with water. However, they do dissolve in milk or alcohol, and so it might be a good idea to wash down spicy foods containing hot peppers with these beverages.

PERCH

Serving Size: 3.5 ounces
Rating: ★★

FAT: 1 gram
CALORIES: 91
SODIUM: 68 mg
B COMPLEX VITAMINS: 10% for B2, 19% for B3
PHOSPHORUS: 18%
POTASSIUM: 230 mg
PROTEIN: 43%

GOOD POINTS

This fish is a very low fat, low calorie, high protein food that contains significant amounts of vitamins B2 and B3, phosphorus and potassium

BAD POINTS

Perch contains quite a lot of sodium. Fish is also commonly implicated in FOOD ALLERGIES.

PERSIMMON

Serving Size: 1 medium (raw, American)
Rating: ★

CALORIES: 32
FAT: 0.1 gram
VITAMIN C: 28%
FIBER: 0.4 mg
POTASSIUM: 78 mg

GOOD POINTS
This low calorie fruit is rich in vitamin C (needed for
healthy gums, teeth, bones, and muscles) and contains good amounts of potassium along with a little
fiber. The American persimmon has nine times as
much vitamin C and twice as much potassium as the
Japanese persimmon.

BAD POINTS
None.

PICKLE

Serving Size: 1 large
Rating: No Stars

	Sour	Kosher	Dill
SODIUM:	1355 mg	581 mg	1428 mg
CALORIES:	10	7	11
FAT:	none	none	none
VITAMIN C:	—	—	10%
FIBER:	0.5 grams	—	0.5 grams
IRON:	18%	—	6%
POTASSIUM:	—	51 mg	200 mg

GOOD POINTS
Sour pickles contain significant amounts of iron,
while dill pickles have a little bit. Dills also contain
quite a lot of potassium and Kosher pickles have a
little. Both sour and dill contain a little fiber. Dills
have a little vitamin C. All are low in calories, but

not good sources for any nutrients considering their major bad point (see below).

BAD POINTS
All types of pickles are extremely high in sodium; sour and dill have twice as much as the Kosher variety.

PIE
(APPLE)
Serving Size: 1/8 pie
Rating: ★

CALORIES: 282
FAT: 11.9 grams
SIMPLE CARBOHYDRATE: 43 grams
SODIUM: 181 mg
B COMPLEX VITAMINS: 9% for B1, 5% for B2, 6% for B3
FIBER: 0.5 grams
IRON: 6%
POTASSIUM: 100 mg

GOOD POINTS
Good old apple pie contains some B vitamins, potassium, iron, and a little fiber. However, the caloric content of this food is so high it's not a great source for any nutrient. When you add ice cream or whipped cream to the top, your waistline will suffer even more!

BAD POINTS
As mentioned, it's very high in calories, as well as simple sugars (bad for your teeth). It also contains significant amounts of saturated fat and sodium. Pie has some GLUTEN in it, which can cause an upset digestive system, anemia, weight loss, bone pain, skin problems, and water retention in people with a condition known as celiac disease.

PINEAPPLE

Serving Size: 1 cup (raw, pieces)
Rating: ★★

CALORIES: 77

FAT: 0.7 grams

SIMPLE CARBOHYDRATE: 19.2 grams

B COMPLEX VITAMINS: 9% for B1, 7% for B6

VITAMIN C: 40%

COPPER: 9%

FIBER: 0.8 grams; much of it is in the form of pectin, which can lower blood cholesterol

MAGNESIUM: 5%

POTASSIUM: 175 mg

GOOD POINTS

Pineapple is a very good, low calorie source of vitamin C (needed for healthy gums, teeth, bones, and muscles), and potassium (needed for proper muscle contractions—including those of the heart—as well as for maintaining the correct fluid balance in the body, helping in the transmission of nerve impulses, and aiding the release of energy from the carbohydrate and protein you eat). It also contains significant amounts of vitamins B1 and B6, potassium, magnesium, copper, and fiber.

BAD POINTS

This fruit is high in simple sugars, which can contribute to tooth decay. It also contains a substance called BROMELAIN, that breaks down protein and can cause IRRITANT DERMATITIS (with symptoms such as lesions and soreness) in anybody who handles it. In addition, pineapple can cause ALLERGIC DERMATITIS in susceptible people.

Fresh pineapple is often treated with SULFITES to protect its vitamin C content and prevent it from darkening in color when exposed to the air. Some people are allergic to these substances, and could develop symptoms such as rashes, watery eyes, and breathing problems.

PISTACHIO

Serving Size: 30 nuts
Rating: ★

CALORIES: 88
FAT: 8 grams
VITAMIN B1: 7%
IRON: 6%
PHOSPHORUS: 8%
POTASSIUM: 147 mg
PROTEIN: 5%

GOOD POINTS

Pistachios are a good source of potassium (needed for proper muscle contractions—including those of the heart—as well as for maintaining the correct fluid balance in the body, helping the transmission of nerve impulses, and for the release of energy from the carbohydrate and protein you eat). They also contain some vitamin B1, iron, phosphorus, and protein.

BAD POINTS

These nuts are high in calories and contain significant amounts of fat—mainly polyunsaturated and monounsaturated. Although these types tend to lower blood cholesterol levels, eating any sort of fat seems to raise your risk of getting breast, uterine, endometrial, ovarian, prostate, and colon cancer. Nuts are often implicated in ALLERGIC REACTIONS.

PIZZA

(WITH CHEESE TOPPING)

Serving Size: ⅛ pie
Rating: ★★

CALORIES: 153
FAT: 5.4 grams
SODIUM: 456 mg
VITAMIN A: 8%
VITAMIN B2: 8%

VITAMIN C: 8%
CALCIUM: 14%
COMPLEX CARBOHYDRATE: 18.4 grams
PHOSPHORUS: 13%
POTASSIUM: 85 mg
PROTEIN: 12%

GOOD POINTS

Pizza is not as bad as you might think: It's a good source of calcium and phosphorus, as well as containing significant amounts of potassium, protein, and vitamins A, B2, and C.

BAD POINTS

It's not that good either: Pizza is high in calories and sodium, as well as containing some fat (mainly saturated from the cheese). If you add extra cheese or toppings you increase the nutrient content as well as the caloric value.

The flour also contains a substance called GLUTEN which can cause an upset digestive system, anemia, weight loss, bone pain, skin problems, and water retention in people with a condition known as celiac disease.

PLANTAIN

Serving Size: 1 cup (slices, cooked)
Rating: ★★★

CALORIES: 179
FAT: 0.3 grams
SIMPLE CARBOHYDRATE: 48 grams
VITAMIN A: 23%
B COMPLEX VITAMINS: 5% for B1, 5% for B2, 6% for B3, 19% for B6, and 10% for folic acid
VITAMIN C: 28%
COPPER: 10%
IRON: 5%
MAGNESIUM: 12%
POTASSIUM: 716 mg

GOOD POINTS

This banana-like fruit is a good source of vitamins A, B6, C, and potassium. It also contains good amounts of magnesium, folic acid, copper, B1, B2, B3, and iron.

BAD POINTS
Plantains are very high in calories and simple sugars (which are bad for your teeth). If you fry them, you'll reduce the vitamin C content and add more calories as well as fat.

PLUM

Serving Size: 1 medium (raw)
Rating: ★

CALORIES: 36

FAT: 0.4 grams

SIMPLE CARBOHYDRATE: 8.6 grams

VITAMIN C: 10%

FIBER: 0.4 grams; some of it is in the form of pectin, which lowers blood cholesterol

POTASSIUM: 113 mg

GOOD POINTS
The plum is a low calorie fruit containing good amounts of vitamin C and potassium, with a little fiber.

BAD POINTS
This fruit has a moderate amount of simple sugars, which can contribute to tooth decay. The pits contain AMYGDALIN, a naturally-occurring substance that breaks down into hydrogen cyanide. While accidentally swallowing the occasional seed is not a problem, taking in a large number of seeds could be hazardous and even a couple of pits could be lethal in a very small child.

POMEGRANATE

Serving Size: 1 medium (raw)
Rating: ★

CALORIES: 104
FAT: 0.5 grams
SIMPLE CARBOHYDRATE: 26.4 grams
B COMPLEX VITAMINS: 8% for B6, 9% for pantothenic acid
VITAMIN C: 15%
POTASSIUM: 399 mg

GOOD POINTS
This fruit contains good amounts of vitamin C, potassium, vitamin B6, and pantothenic acid.

BAD POINTS
The pomegranate is high in calories and simple sugars.

RAISINS

Serving Size: 1 ounce
Rating: ★

CALORIES: 81
FAT: 0.2 grams
SIMPLE CARBOHYDRATE: 25 grams
COPPER: 5%
FIBER: 2.2 grams; most of it is in the form of pectin, which can lower blood cholesterol
IRON: 7%
POTASSIUM: 250 mg

GOOD POINTS
Raisins are an excellent source of potassium, needed for proper muscle contractions (including those of the heart), for maintaining the correct fluid balance in the body, to help the transmission of nerve impulses, and for the release of energy from the carbohydrate and protein you eat. They also contain fiber, iron,

copper, and vitamin B6. They are neither high nor low in calories.

BAD POINTS
Raisins are high in simple sugars which stick to the teeth when you eat them, thereby increasing your risk of tooth decay. They may be sprayed with SULFITES to preserve them. Some people are allergic to these substances, and could develop symptoms such as rashes, watery eyes, and breathing problems. Dark raisins also contain a substance called TYRAMINE, which can be dangerous when consumed by someone who is taking monoamine oxidase inhibitors (MAOI's), a group of antidepressant medications.

POPCORN
Serving Size: 1 cup
Rating: ★

CALORIES: 23; with fat added 41
FAT: 0.3 grams; with fat added 2 grams
COMPLEX CARBOHYDRATE: 10.7 grams
FIBER: 0.3 grams
MAGNESIUM: 6%

GOOD POINTS
This popular low-calorie snack contains a little magnesium and some fiber.

BAD POINTS
Plain popcorn really has no bad points, but if you add butter or salt to it, you can make it higher in calories, with plenty of saturated fat and sodium. Cheese-flavored popcorn is similarly higher in calories and fat than the plain kind.

PORK

Serving Size: 1 medium loin chop
(cooked)
Rating: ★★

CALORIES: 314
CHOLESTEROL: 72 mg
FAT: 22.5 grams
SODIUM: 84 mg
B COMPLEX VITAMINS: 44% for B1, 12% for B2, 29% for B3, 16% for B6 17% for B12, and 10% for pantothenic acid
COPPER: 9%
IRON: 7-19%
MAGNESIUM: 7%
PHOSPHORUS: 23%
POTASSIUM: 380 mg
PROTEIN: 58%
ZINC: 19%

GOOD POINTS

Pork is an excellent source of protein, potassium, and B vitamins, and a good source of zinc and phosphorus. In addition, it contains substantial amounts of iron, copper, and magnesium.

BAD POINTS

Pork is high in calories and fat. The fat is about half saturated and half monounsaturated, which means that it has less saturated fat than you would find in beef or veal. However, eating any type of fat seems to increase your risk of getting certain types of cancers. Pork contains about the same amount of cholesterol as beef, as well as significant quantities of sodium.

It should always be cooked thoroughly as it can contain a parasitic worm called TRICHINOSIS. If eaten alive this will cause symptoms similar to the flu—aches, fever, and dizziness. Many Americans (4% of the population) carry this parasite but few ever show any symptoms or develop the disease. If left untreated, the disease can result in death.

POTATO, SWEET

Serving Size: 1 small (baked)
Rating: ★★★

CALORIES: 141
FAT: 0.2 grams
SIMPLE CARBOHYDRATE: 32.5 grams
VITAMIN A: 60–160%
B COMPLEX VITAMINS: 6% for B1, 7% for B6, 6% for folic acid, and 6% for pantothenic acid
VITAMIN C: 37%
COPPER: 8%
VITAMIN E: 20%
FIBER: .9 grams
IRON: 5%
PHOSPHORUS: 6%
POTASSIUM: 300 mg

GOOD POINTS

Sweet potatoes are an excellent source of vitamin A as carotene (an anti-cancer nutrient); the darker the color the higher the A content. They also contain a lot of vitamin C—needed for healthy gums, teeth, bones, and muscles—in addition to potassium, vitamin E, the B vitamins, iron, copper, phosphorus, and a little fiber.

BAD POINTS

Sweet potatoes are high in calories due to their carbohydrate content. The sweeter the potato, the higher the level of simple sugars. They also contain a **CYANIDE COMPOUND** which is converted into hydrogen cyanide as the potato is heated. Pierce the potato or leave the lid off the saucepan when cooking to allow the cyanide gas to escape into the air.

POTATO, WHITE

Serving Size: 1 medium (baked)
Rating: ★★

CALORIES: 95

FAT: 0.1 grams

B COMPLEX VITAMINS: 7% for B1, 9% for B3, 9% for B6

VITAMIN C: 33%

COPPER: 8%

COMPLEX CARBOHYDRATE: 21.1 grams

FIBER: 0.6 grams

MAGNESIUM: 6%

PHOSPHORUS: 7%

POTASSIUM: 503 mg

GOOD POINTS

Potatoes are an excellent source of vitamin C (needed for healthy gums, teeth, bones, and muscles) and potassium (needed for proper muscle contractions, for maintaining the correct fluid balance in the body, to help the transmission of nerve impulses, and for the release of energy from the carbohydrate and protein you eat). They also contain significant amounts of several B vitamins, copper, magnesium, phosphorus, as well as a little fiber. They can be cooked in a variety of ways and complete any main course.

BAD POINTS

This vegetable is moderately (though not excessively) high in calories. You shouldn't eat potatoes with green spots or sprouting eyes as they contain a lot of SOLANINE, which acts as a nerve poison.

POTATO CHIPS
Serving Size: 1 ounce
Rating: ★

CALORIES: 159
FAT: 11 grams
SODIUM: 80 mg
B COMPLEX VITAMINS: 7% for B3, 14% for B6
VITAMIN C: 8%
COMPLEX CARBOHYDRATE: 14 grams
VITAMIN E: 10%
FIBER: 0.45 grams
POTASSIUM: 316 mg

GOOD POINTS
Potato chips are very good sources of potassium, and contain significant amounts of vitamins B3, B6, E, C, as well as a little fiber.

BAD POINTS
They are high in calories, sodium, and fat. Although the fat is mainly polyunsaturated and monunsaturated and tends to lower blood cholesterol levels, it can still be a problem: Eating any sort of fat seems to raise your risk of getting breast, uterine, endometrial, ovarian, prostrate, and colon cancer.

PRETZEL
Serving Size: 1 ounce
Rating: No stars

CALORIES: 111
FAT: 1 gram
SODIUM: 451 mg
VITAMIN B1: 6%
VITAMIN B2: 6%
COMPLEX CARBOHYDRATE: 22.4 grams

GOOD POINTS
Pretzels contain some vitamin B1 and B3—and that's about it!

Pretzels are high in calories and very high in sodium—not advisable for waistline or salt watchers. They also contain a substance called GLUTEN which can cause an upset digestive system, anemia, weight loss, bone pain, skin problems, and water retention in people with a condition known as celiac disease.

PRUNE

Serving Size: 5
Rating: ★★★

CALORIES: 100
FAT: 0.2 grams
SIMPLE CARBOHYDRATE: 25 grams
VITAMIN A: 17%
B COMPLEX VITAMINS: 6% for B2, 7% for B6
COPPER: 8%
IRON: 8%
PHOSPHORUS: 5%
POTASSIUM: 430 mg

GOOD POINTS

Prunes contain a natural laxative (that speeds up the muscular contractions in the intestine and pushes its contents through more quickly), in addition to being high in fiber. These two factors combined make prunes excellent for preventing constipation; by doing so, they possibly reduce your risk for getting cancer of the colon and rectum. They are also very good sources of vitamin A (as carotene) and potassium, and contain significant amounts of copper, iron, vitamins B2 and B6, and phosphorus.

BAD POINTS

Prunes are quite high in calories because of their simple sugar content. Also, prunes tend to stick to the teeth—like all dried fruit—making them a high risk food for tooth decay. Dried prunes are often treated with SULFITES to prevent them from darkening in color. Some people are allergic to these substances and could develop symptoms such as rashes, watery eyes and breathing problems.

PRUNE JUICE

Serving Size: 1 cup
Rating: ★★

CALORIES: 181
FAT: 1 gram
SIMPLE CARBOHYDRATE: 44.7 grams
B COMPLEX VITAMINS: 11% for B2, 10% for B3
VITAMIN C: 18%
COPPER: 9%
IRON: 17%
MAGNESIUM: 9%
PHOSPHORUS: 6%
POTASSIUM: 706 mg

GOOD POINTS
Prune juice is an excellent source of potassium (needed for proper muscle contractions, for maintaining the correct fluid balance in the body, to help the transmission of nerve impulses, and for the release of energy from the carbohydrate and protein you eat), and a very good source of vitamin C and iron. It also contains vitamins B2, B3, copper, iron, magnesium, and phosphorus. Prune juice, like prunes, contains a natural laxative that speeds up the contractions of the muscles in the intestines and propels its contents through to the outside more quickly than usual, thereby preventing constipation and possibly offering protection in this way against cancers of the rectum and colon.

BAD POINTS
Prune juice is very high in calories and simple sugars (which can increase your risk for tooth decay).

PUDDING, CHOCOLATE

Serving Size: 1/2 cup (from instant mix)
Rating: ★★

CALORIES: 178
CHOLESTEROL: 17 mg
FAT: 4.6 grams (if whole milk is used)
SIMPLE CARBOHYDRATE: 31.6 grams
SODIUM: 495 mg (if from instant mix)
B COMPLEX VITAMINS: 12% for B2, 7% for B12
CALCIUM: 15%
MAGNESIUM: 8%
PHOSPHORUS: 39%
POTASSIUM: 208 mg
PROTEIN: 10%

GOOD POINTS

One of the favorite desserts for children, chocolate pudding contains a lot of phosphorus and is a good source of protein, vitamin B2, potassium, and calcium. It also has magnesium and vitamin B12.

BAD POINTS

Chocolate pudding is very high in calories and simple sugars (which can contribute to tooth decay). It contains some fat and cholesterol; the amount is dependent on the kind of milk used to make the pudding (see MILK). Instant mix is very high in sodium; the non-instant type has half as much.

Because of the lactose it contains and the milk used, as well as the chocolate, ALLERGIC REACTION and LACTOSE INTOLERANCE could be a problem for susceptible people.

Chocolate contains a substance called PHENYL-ETHYLAMINE that can cause headaches in people taking a class of antidepressant drugs called MAO inhibitors, by raising blood pressure about 12 hours after they eat the chocolate.

PUDDING, VANILLA

Serving Size: 1/2 cup (from instant mix)
Rating: ★★

CALORIES: 177
CHOLESTEROL: 17 mg
FAT: 4.3 grams (if whole milk is used)
SIMPLE CARBOHYDRATE: 30.9 grams
SODIUM: 422 mg (if from instant mix)
B COMPLEX VITAMINS: 12% for B2, 10% for B12
CALCIUM: 15%
POTASSIUM: 189 mg
PROTEIN: 9%

GOOD POINTS
Vanilla pudding is a very good source of phosphorus and a good source of calcium, vitamins B2, B12, potassium, and protein.

BAD POINTS
It's very high in calories, simple sugars, and sodium (although the non-instant mix has half as much). It also contains significant amounts of fat and cholesterol, depending on which type of milk is used (see MILK). Because of the milk, FOOD ALLERGIES and LACTOSE INTOLERANCE could be a problem for susceptible people.

PUMPKIN

Serving Size: 2/5 cup (canned)
Rating: ★★★★

CALORIES: 33
FAT: 0.2 grams
VITAMIN A: 400–700%
VITAMIN C: 8%
COPPER: 6%
FIBER: 1.4 grams; some of it is in the form of pectin, which lowers blood cholesterol
MAGNESIUM: 6%
POTASSIUM: 219 mg

GOOD POINTS

This festive vegetable, popular for pie filling, is an extremely rich source of vitamin A (as carotene), needed for healthy skin, hair, and eyes, and to help protect the body from respiratory and gastrointestinal tract cancer. Pumpkin is low in calories and contains potassium, vitamin C, magnesium, copper, and fiber. (Pumpkin seeds are also rich in nutrients with good amounts of vitamin E, iron, vitamin B1, protein, and fiber.)

BAD POINTS

None.

QUAIL

Serving Size: 3.5 ounces
Rating: ★★★★

CALORIES: 134

FAT: 4.5 grams

SODIUM: 51 mg

B COMPLEX VITAMINS: 19% for B1, 17% for B2, and 31% for B3

VITAMIN C: 12%

COPPER: 30%

IRON: 25%

PHOSPHORUS: 31%

POTASSIUM: 237 mg

PROTEIN: 48%

GOOD POINTS

This wise poultry choice is an excellent source of protein, iron, copper, phosphorus and vitamin B3. It contains good amounts of B1 and B2, potassium and vitamin C. And if all that isn't enough, it's also low in calories.

BAD POINTS

Quail contains a little sodium and a little fat (about half saturated and half unsaturated).

RABBIT

Serving Size: 3.5 ounces
Rating: ★★

CALORIES: 179
CHOLESTEROL: 70
FAT: 7.7 grams
B COMPLEX VITAMINS: 16% for B2, 43% for B3, 25% for B6, and 200% for B12
IRON: 11%
MAGNESIUM: 6%
PHOSPHORUS: 20%
POTASSIUM: 210 mg
PROTEIN: 60%

GOOD POINTS
Rabbit is an excellent source of vitamins B3, B6, B12, and protein, as well as having good amounts of potassium, phosphorus, iron, B2, and some magnesium. It contains neither a small nor great amount of calories.

BAD POINTS
It is quite high in cholesterol and fat (about half saturated and half unsaturated).

RADISH

Serving Size: 10 small
Rating: ★★

CALORIES: 7
FAT: 0.2
VITAMIN C: 43%
COMPLEX CARBOHYDRATE: 3.6 grams
FIBER: 0.7 grams
IRON: 6%
POTASSIUM: 322 mg

GOOD POINTS
These low-calorie vegetables, often added to salads, are an excellent source of vitamin C (needed for

healthy gums, teeth, bones, and muscles) and a good source of potassium (needed for proper muscle contractions, for maintaining the correct fluid balance in the body, to help the transmission of nerve impulses, and for the release of energy from the carbohydrate and protein you eat). They also contain some iron and fiber.

BAD POINTS
All cruciferous (belonging to the cabbage family) vegetables like radishes contain GOITROGENS—substances that hamper the production of thyroid hormones by the thyroid gland. This can cause an enlargement of the gland (goiter) in an attempt by the body to compensate for the reduced hormone production by increasing the amount of tissue available. However, people with healthy thyroids would have to eat a very large amount of these vegetables before they would have any kind of problem. This is only of concern for those with sluggish thyroid glands.

RASPBERRIES

Serving Size: 1 cup
Rating: ★★

CALORIES: 61
FAT: 0.7 grams
SIMPLE CARBOHYDRATE: 14.2 grams
B COMPLEX VITAMINS: 6% for B2, 6% for B3
VITAMIN C: 50%
COPPER: 12%
FIBER: 3.7 grams; most of it is in the form of pectin, which lowers blood cholesterol
MAGNESIUM: 6%
POTASSIUM: 187 mg

GOOD POINTS
This delicious, low-calorie fruit is an excellent source of vitamin C—needed for healthy gums, teeth, bones, and muscles—and a good source of fiber, for the prevention of constipation and other related

gastrointestinal disorders. It also contains significant amounts of copper and potassium, as well as some magnesium and B vitamins.

BAD POINTS
Raspberries are quite high in simple sugars, which can contribute to tooth decay.

RAVIOLI
(BEEF)

Serving Size: 7.5 ounces (one portion)
Rating: ★★

CALORIES: 210

FAT: 8 grams

SODIUM: 990 mg

VITAMIN A: 37%

B COMPLEX VITAMINS: 11% for B1, 10% for B2, 14% for B3

COMPLEX CARBOHYDRATE: 34 grams

IRON: 13%

PHOSPHORUS: 11%

POTASSIUM: 162 mg

PROTEIN: 18%

GOOD POINTS
Beef ravioli is a very good source of vitamin A as carotene; vitamin A is needed for healthy skin, hair, and eyes, and to help protect the body from respiratory and gastrointestinal tract cancer. Ravioli is also a good source of protein, several B vitamins, potassium, phosphorus, and iron.

BAD POINTS
Beef ravioli is high in calories and sodium, and has significant amounts of fat. It also contains a substance called GLUTEN which can cause an upset digestive system, anemia, weight loss, bone pain, skin problems, and water retention in people with a condition known as celiac disease.

REDFISH (OCEAN PERCH)

Serving Size: 3.5 ounces (raw)
Rating: ★★★

CALORIES: 88
FAT: 1.1 grams
SODIUM: 79 mg
B COMPLEX VITAMINS: 7% for B1, 5% for B2, and
   10% for B3
IODINE: 10%
IRON: 6%
MAGNESIUM: 8%
PHOSPHORUS: 21%
POTASSIUM: 269 mg
PROTEIN: 40%

GOOD POINTS

Redfish is a very good, low-calorie source of protein that is extremely low in fat. It also contains good amounts of phosphorus, potassium, vitamin B3, iodine, and magnesium, in addition to some B1, B2, and iron. Health-conscious eaters should try to get fish like redfish into their diets at least three times a week.

BAD POINTS

About the only bad thing you can say about redfish is that it contains a little sodium.

RELISH

Serving Size: 1 tablespoon
Rating: No stars

CALORIE: 53
FAT: 0.1 gram
SIMPLE CARBOHYDRATE: 13.6 grams

GOOD POINTS

None; relishes do not contain significant amounts of any essential nutrient.

BAD POINTS

They do contain significant amounts of simple carbohydrates (which can contribute to tooth decay) and
calories.

RHUBARB

*Serving Size: ¹/₂ cup (stewed without
sugar)*
Rating: ★★

CALORIES: 10
FAT: 0.1 grams
VITAMIN C: 13%
COPPER: 6%
FIBER: 2.4 grams
POTASSIUM: 400 mg

GOOD POINTS

This tart, low-calorie fruit is a very good source of
potassium, needed for proper muscle contractions
(including those of the heart), for maintaining the
correct fluid balance in the body, to help the
transmission of nerve impulses, and for the release of
energy from the carbohydrate and protein you eat. It
is also a good source of vitamin C and fiber, and
contains some copper. Most people eat it stewed or
use it as a pie filling.

BAD POINTS

Rhubarb contains TANNINS, chemicals which tend
to cause CONSTIPATION. If you add sugar to the
rhubarb this will, of course, raise the calorie value.

RICE

(WHITE, ENRICHED)

Serving Size: ⁴/₅ cup (cooked)
Rating: ★★

CALORIES: 164
FAT: 0.1 grams
SODIUM: 561 mg
B COMPLEX VITAMINS: 11% for B1, 8% for B3
COMPLEX CARBOHYDRATE: 36 grams
IRON: 8%
PROTEIN: 5%

GOOD POINTS

Enriched white rice contains a good amount of the B vitamins (needed for getting energy from your food, keeping your eyes and skin healthy, and for many reactions in the brain). It also contains iron and protein.

BAD POINTS

This type of rice is high in calories and sodium.

(NOTE: Brown rice has about the same nutrient content, except for the fact that it is not high in sodium. White rice that is not enriched has a much lower nutrient content but is also high in sodium.)

SAFFLOWER SEEDS

Serving Size: 1 ounce
Rating: ★

CALORIES: 172
FAT: 16.7 grams
VITAMIN E: 67%
PROTEIN: 8%

GOOD POINTS

Safflower seeds are an extremely rich source of vitamin E, which has an important role to play in protecting our cell membranes from wear and tear, and helping to prevent the formation of free radicals (substances believed to be a cause of cancer). The seeds also contain some protein.

BAD POINTS
They're nice to nibble on, but safflower seeds are high in fat and calories. Even though the fat is almost entirely polyunsaturated and monounsaturated and tends to lower blood cholesterol levels, there is still some cause for concern; eating any sort of fat seems to raise your risk of getting breast, uterine, endometrial, ovarian, prostate, and colon cancer.

SALAD DRESSING
Serving Size: 1 tablespoon
Rating: Sorry, no stars

CALORIES: Blue, 84; French 67; Italian, 69; Russian, 76; Thousand Island, 59; Vinegar and Oil, 72

FAT: Blue, 9.1 grams; French, 6.4 grams; Italian, 7.1 grams; Russian, 7.8 grams; Thousand Island, 5.6 grams; Vinegar and Oil, 8.0 grams

SODIUM: Blue, 214 mg; French, 214 mg; Italian, 116 mg; Russian, 133 mg; Thousand Island, 109 mg; Vinegar and Oil 0.

GOOD POINTS
None.

BAD POINTS
Any type of salad dressing contains significant amounts of calories, sodium (except for vinegar and oil) and fat (mainly polyunsaturated and monounsaturated). Although this type tends to lower blood cholesterol levels, eating any sort of fat seems to raise your risk of getting breast, uterine, endometrial, ovarian, prostate, and colon cancer.

SALAMI

Serving Size: 1 slice
Rating: ★

CALORIES: 58
CHOLESTEROL: 14 mg
FAT: 4.6 grams
SODIUM: 266 mg
VITAMIN B12: 19%
POTASSIUM: 52 mg
PROTEIN: 8%

GOOD POINTS

Salami contains a good amount of vitamin B12 and significant amounts of protein and potassium. However, it is not a great source for these nutrients because of its bad points.

BAD POINTS

It is high in fat (mainly saturated), cholesterol, calories, and sodium. This is bad for people watching their salt intake, weight, or arteries.

SALMON

Serving Size: 3.5 ounces (cooked)
Rating: ★★★

CHOLESTEROL: 80 mg
FAT: 13 grams
SODIUM: 110 mg
B COMPLEX VITAMINS: 13% for B1, 6% for B2, 35% for B3, 42% for B6, 100% for B12, 7% for folic acid, and 18% for pantothenic acid
CALORIES: 197
IODINE: 10%
MAGNESIUM: 7%
PHOSPHORUS: 30%
POTASSIUM: 330 mg
PROTEIN: 44%

GOOD POINTS

Salmon is an excellent source of vitamin B3, B6, B12, protein, phosphorus, and potassium. It also contains iodine, pantothenic acid, vitamin B1, B2, magnesium, and folic acid. Salmon has one of the highest contents of the omega-3 fatty acids, believed to lower blood cholesterol. It is neither very high nor low in calories.

BAD POINTS

Salmon is a very high fat fish; the darker the color the higher the fat content. While the fat is mainly polyunsaturated and monounsaturated and tends to lower blood cholesterol levels, eating any sort of fat seems to raise your risk of getting breast, uterine, endometrial, ovarian, prostate, and colon cancer. Salmon also contains quite a lot of cholesterol. Fish is often implicated in FOOD ALLERGIES.

SALT

Serving Size: 1 teaspoon
Rating: ★

SODIUM: 2300 mg
IODINE: 100%
CALORIES: none
FAT: none

GOOD POINTS

If the salt is iodized it contains at least 100% of the RDA for this nutrient, needed for the manufacture of thyroid hormone.

BAD POINTS

Salt is sodium chloride and therefore extremely high in sodium.

SARDINES

Serving Size: 8 medium (canned in oil)
Rating: ★★★

CALORIES: 217

CHOLESTEROL: 100 mg

FAT: 13.6 grams

SODIUM: 650 mg

B COMPLEX VITAMINS: 21% for B2, 41% for B3, 24% for B6, 466% for B12, 5% for pantothenic acid

VITAMIN D: 75%

CALCIUM: 55% (if you eat the bones)

COPPER: 10%

IODINE: 10%

IRON: 16%

MAGNESIUM: 13%

PHOSPHORUS: 52% (if you eat the bones)

POTASSIUM: 53%

PROTEIN: 53%

ZINC: 20%

GOOD POINTS

These small fish, usually eaten for lunch or as appetizers, are a real nutrient storehouse! They are an excellent source of vitamin B3, B12, D, protein, potassium, calcium, and phosphorus. They also contain good amounts of B2, B6, zinc, iron, iodine, copper, and magnesium, in addition to some pantothenic acid. Sardines contain quite a lot of the omega-3 fatty acids (about half as much as salmon), believed to lower blood cholesterol levels.

BAD POINTS

Sardines contain quite a lot of cholesterol and fat. Although the fat is polyunsaturated and monounsaturated and tends to lower blood cholesterol levels, eating any sort of fat seems to raise your risk of getting breast, uterine, endometrial, ovarian, prostate, and colon cancer. They are also very high in sodium. Fish is often implicated in FOOD ALLERGIES.

Sausage, Smoked Beef

Serving Size: 1
Rating: ★

CALORIES: 160
CHOLESTEROL: 30 mg
FAT: 14.6 grams
SODIUM: 455 mg
B COMPLEX VITAMINS: 7% for B3, 14% for B12
VITAMIN C: 8%
POTASSIUM: 78 mg
PROTEIN: 17%
ZINC: 8%

GOOD POINTS
This type of sausage is a good source of potassium and vitamin B12, and also contains some C, B3, protein, and zinc.

BAD POINTS
Sausage contains a lot of saturated fat and some cholesterol. It is high in calories and sodium. This is not a great choice for health and weight conscious eaters.

Sausage, Italian

Serving Size: 1 link (cooked)
Rating: ★

CALORIES: 216
CHOLESTEROL: 52 mg
FAT: 17.2 grams
SODIUM: 618 mg
B COMPLEX VITAMINS: 28% for B1, 9% for B2, 14% for B3, 11% for B6 and 15% for B12
IRON: 6%
PHOSPHORUS: 11%
POTASSIUM: 204 mg
PROTEIN: 30%
ZINC: 11%

GOOD POINTS
Italian sausage is a very good source of protein and vitamin B1, and also contains B2, B3, B6, B12, phosphorus, potassium, and zinc, as well as some iron.

BAD POINTS
It is very high in calories, fat (mainly saturated), cholesterol, and sodium. This is not a great choice for health and weight conscious eaters.

SAUSAGE, LIVERWURST

Serving Size: 1 slice
Rating: ★

CALORIES: 59
CHOLESTEROL: 28 mg
FAT: 5.1 grams
B COMPLEX VITAMINS: 257% for B12, 5% for pantothenic acid
IRON: 6%
PROTEIN: 6%

GOOD POINTS
Liverwurst sausage is an excellent source of vitamin B12, and contains some protein, pantothenic acid, and iron. Unlike other types of sausage, it is not high in calories.

BAD POINTS
It is high in saturated fat and cholesterol. In addition, it contains a substance called TYRAMINE, which can be very dangerous when consumed by someone who is on monoamine oxidase inhibitors (MAOI's), a group of antidepressant medications.

SAUSAGE, PORK
Serving Size: 1
Rating: ★

CALORIES: 206
CHOLESTEROL: 43 mg
FAT: 18.6 grams
SODIUM: 615 mg
B COMPLEX VITAMINS: 18% for B1, 6% for B2, 11% for B3, 9% for B6 and 9% for B12
PHOSPHORUS: 10%
POTASSIUM: 127 mg
PROTEIN: 20%
ZINC: 10%

GOOD POINTS
Pork sausage is a good source of protein, vitamin B1, B3, B6, B12, phosphorus, potassium, zinc, and some B2.

BAD POINTS
It is very high in fat, calories, cholesterol, and sodium. Even though the fat is mainly polyunsaturated and monounsaturated, and tends to lower blood cholesterol levels, eating any sort of fat seems to raise your risk of getting breast, uterine, endometrial, ovarian, prostate, and colon cancer.

SCALLION
Serving Size: 5 medium (raw)
Rating: ★★

CALORIES: 45
FAT: 0.3 grams
SIMPLE CARBOHYDRATE: 10.5 grams
VITAMIN C: 42%
FIBER: 1 gram
POTASSIUM: 231 mg

GOOD POINTS
Scallions are a very good source of vitamin C (needed for healthy gums, teeth, bones, and muscles) and a

good source of potassium (needed for proper muscle contractions, for maintaining the correct fluid balance in the body, to help the transmission of nerve impulses, and for the release of energy from the carbohydrate and protein you eat). They also contain some fiber.

BAD POINTS
Scallions have some simple sugars, which can contribute to tooth decay. You can suffer from HALITOSIS (BAD BREATH) because of the sulfur compounds they contain.

SCALLOPS
(BAY AND SEA)

Serving Size: 3.5 ounces (steamed)
Rating: ★★

CALORIES: 81
CHOLESTEROL: 35 mg
FAT: 0.7 grams
SODIUM: 255 mg
VITAMIN B3: 7%
IODINE: 10%
IRON: 10%
PHOSPHORUS: 20%
POTASSIUM: 396 mg
PROTEIN: 34%

GOOD POINTS
Scallops are a very good source of protein (required for the growth and maintenance of all your body tissues) and potassium (needed for proper muscle contractions, for maintaining the correct fluid balance in the body, to help the transmission of nerve impulses, and for the release of energy from the carbohydrate and protein you eat). They are low in calories, and contain good amounts of phosphorus, iron, iodine, and some vitamin B3.

BAD POINTS
Scallops contain some cholesterol, but not significant amounts of any other type of fat. They are also quite

high in sodium. Seafood is implicated in FOOD ALLERGIES.

Sesame Seeds

Serving Size: 1 ounce
Rating: ★

CALORIES: 167
FAT: 15.5 grams
B COMPLEX VITAMINS: 14% for B1, 7% for B3
FIBER: 0.9 grams
IRON: 12%
MAGNESIUM: 25%
PHOSPHORUS: 22%
POTASSIUM: 117 mg
PROTEIN: 7.5 grams
ZINC: 19%

GOOD POINTS
These seeds are a very good source of magnesium, phosphorus and zinc, and a good source of protein, vitamin B1, iron, and potassium. They also contain some vitamin B3 and fiber.

BAD POINTS
They are high in calories and fat. Although the fat is manly polyunsaturated and monounsaturated and tends to lower blood cholesterol levels, eating any sort of fat seems to raise your risk of getting breast, uterine, endometrial, ovarian, prostate, and colon cancer.

Shallots

Serving Size: 1.75 ounces (raw).
Rating: ★

CALORIES: 36
FAT: none
SIMPLE CARBOHYDRATE: 8.4 grams
VITAMIN C: 7%

FIBER: 0.4 grams
POTASSIUM: 167 mg

GOOD POINTS

These small onions, used for flavoring, are very low in calories and a good source of potassium (needed for proper muscle contractions, for maintaining the correct fluid balance in the body, to help the transmission of nerve impulses, and for the release of energy from the carbohydrate and protein you eat). They also contain some vitamin C and fiber.

BAD POINTS

They contain some simple carbohydrate, which can contribute to tooth decay.

SHRIMP

Serving Size: 3.5 ounces
Rating: ★★

CALORIES: 91
CHOLESTEROL: 200 mg
FAT: 1.5 grams
SODIUM: 14 mg
B COMPLEX VITAMINS: 16% for B3, 5% for B6
CALCIUM: 6%
COPPER: 40%
IODINE: 24%
IRON: 9%
MAGNESIUM: 11%
PHOSPHORUS: 17%
POTASSIUM: 220 mg
PROTEIN: 42%
ZINC: 35%

GOOD POINTS

Shrimp are an excellent source of protein, zinc, and copper, and a very good source of iodine. They also contain B vitamins, phosphorus, magnesium, potassium, calcium, and iron, and are low in calories. However, before you choose this food for its impressive nutrient value, it might be wise to check out its bad points below.

BAD POINTS

Shrimp are very high in cholesterol and contain a significant amount of sodium. Shellfish are often implicated in FOOD ALLERGIES. In addition, shrimp may be treated with SULFITES to prevent darkening. Some people are allergic to these substances, and could develop symptoms such as rashes, watery eyes, and breathing problems.

SNAPPER (RED)

Serving Size: 3.5 ounces
Rating: ★★★

CALORIES: 93
FAT: 1.2 grams
SODIUM: 67 mg
VITAMIN B1: 11%
IODINE: 10%
PHOSPHORUS: 21%
POTASSIUM: 323 mg
PROTEIN: 44%

GOOD POINTS

Red snapper is an excellent source of good quality protein, required for the growth and maintenance of all your body tissues. It is very low in fat and calories, and a good source of potassium, phosphorus, vitamin B1, and iodine. Health-conscious eaters should try to get fishes like red snapper into their diets at least three times a week.

BAD POINTS

Red snapper contains some sodium. Fish are often implicated in FOOD ALLERGIES.

SOFT DRINKS

Serving Size: 12 fluid ounces
Rating: Sorry, no stars

CALORIES: Club soda, none; Cola, 159; Ginger ale, 113; Orange drink, 179; Root beer, 163

FAT: Club soda, none; Cola, none; Ginger ale, none; Orange drink, none; Root beer, none

SIMPLE CARBOHYDRATE: Club soda, none; Cola, 40.7 grams; Ginger ale, 29 grams; Orange drink, 45.8 grams, Root beer, 42.2 grams

SODIUM: Club soda, 78 mg; Cola, 20 mg; Ginger ale, 30 mg; Orange drink, 52 mg; Root beer, 49

GOOD POINTS
None, except when vitamin C is added to the beverage.

BAD POINTS
Soft drinks contain a lot of calories, with a high simple sugar content (bad for your teeth). Some sodas contain significant amounts of sodium and a lot contain CAFFEINE. The diet beverages often contain ASPARTAME as an artificial sweetener, which breaks down into aspartic acid, phenylalanine, and methanol in the stomach. The phenylalanine may cause MOOD CHANGES in susceptible people.

SOLE

Serving Size: 3.5 ounces (steamed)
Rating: ★★★

CALORIES: 91
CHOLESTEROL: 60 mg
FAT: 0.7 grams
SODIUM: 120 mg
B COMPLEX VITAMINS: 6% for B1, 5% for B2, 18% for B3, 17% for B12
COPPER: 6%

IODINE: 10%
MAGNESIUM: 5%
PHOSPHORUS: 25%
POTASSIUM: 280 mg
PROTEIN: 46%

GOOD POINTS
Sole is an excellent source of protein, required for the growth and maintenance of all your body tissues. It also contains good amounts of B vitamins, potassium, phosphorus and iodine, along with some copper and magnesium. It is low in calories and fat.

BAD POINTS
Sole contains some cholesterol and sodium. Fish is often implicated in FOOD ALLERGIES.

SOUP, THICK, CHICKEN
Serving Size: 1 cup
Rating: ★★

CALORIES: 178
CHOLESTEROL: 30 mg
FAT: 6.6 grams
SODIUM: 887 mg
VITAMIN A: 26%
B COMPLEX VITAMINS: 6% for B1, 10% for B2, 22% for B3
COMPLEX CARBOHYDRATE: 17.3 grams
COPPER: 13%
IRON: 10%
PHOSPHORUS: 11%
POTASSIUM: 176 mg
PROTEIN: 28%
ZINC: 7%

GOOD POINTS
This type of soup is a very good source of protein, vitamin A, B3, and a good source of B2, phosphorus, potassium, iron, and copper. It also contains some B1 and zinc.

BAD POINTS

It's very high in sodium, contains some fat (mainly saturated and monounsaturated), and cholesterol. It is also quite high in calories; the thicker the soup, the higher the caloric content.

SOUP, THICK, VEGETABLE

Serving Size: 1 cup
Rating: ★★

CALORIES: 167
FAT: 4.8 grams
SODIUM: 1010 mg
VITAMIN A: 118%
B COMPLEX VITAMINS: 6% for B3, 9.5% for B6
VITAMIN C: 10%
CALCIUM: 6%
COMPLEX CARBOHYDRATE: 19.0 grams
COPPER: 12%
FIBER: 1.2 grams
IRON: 9%
PHOSPHORUS: 7%
POTASSIUM: 396 mg
PROTEIN: 5%
ZINC: 21%

GOOD POINTS

It is an excellent source of vitamin A as carotene, needed for healthy skin, hair, and eyes, and to help protect the body from respiratory and gastrointestinal tract cancer. It's a very good source of potassium and zinc, and contains copper, vitamin C, iron, phosphorus, calcium, vitamin B3, B6, fiber, and protein.

BAD POINTS

It's extremely high in sodium, and contains some fat.

SOUP, TOMATO

Serving Size: 1 cup
Rating:★★

CALORIES: 86

FAT: 2.5 grams

SODIUM: 872 mg

VITAMIN A: 14%

B COMPLEX VITAMINS: 6% for B1, 7% for B3, 6% for B6

VITAMIN C: 112%

COMPLEX CARBOHYDRATE: 16.6 grams

COPPER: 13%

IRON: 10%

POTASSIUM: 263 mg

GOOD POINTS
Tomato soup is an excellent source of vitamin C, needed for healthy gums, teeth, bones, and muscles. It is also low in calories and contains good amounts of vitamin A (as carotene), iron, copper, B1 and B3.

BAD POINTS
It's very high in sodium.

SOY SAUCE

Serving Size: 1 tablespoon
Rating:★

FAT: none

SODIUM: 1029 mg

POTASSIUM: 64 mg

GOOD POINTS
Soy sauce, traditionally served to flavor oriental food, contains a little potassium. It is very useful when eating raw fish, as in Japanese food, since it deactivates an enzyme that would normally destroy the nutrients (such as vitamin B1) in the fish.

BAD POINTS:

It's extremely high in sodium. It is also extremely high in a substance called TYRAMINE, which can be very dangerous when consumed by someone who is taking monoamine oxidase inhibitors (MAOI's), a group of antidepressant medications.

SPAGHETTI

Serving Size: 1 cup (cooked)
Rating: ★ ★

CALORIES: 210

FAT: 1.1 grams

B COMPLEX VITAMINS: 17% for B1, 9% for B2, 10% for B3

COMPLEX CARBOHYDRATE: 44 grams

IRON: 9%

MAGNESIUM: 7%

PHOSPHORUS: 10%

POTASSIUM: 115 mg

PROTEIN: 11%

GOOD POINTS

It's a very good source of protein, vitamin B1, B3, phosphorus. It also contains vitamin B2, magnesium, iron, and potassium.

BAD POINTS

As you might imagine, spaghetti is pretty high in calories. It also contains a substance called GLUTEN, that can cause an upset digestive system, anemia, weight loss, bone pain, skin problems, and water retention in people with a condition known as celiac disease.

SPINACH

Serving Size: ¹/₂ cup (boiled)
Rating:★★★

CALORIES: 21
FAT: 0.2 grams
SODIUM: 120 mg
VITAMIN A: 120%
B COMPLEX VITAMINS: 5% for B1, 9% for B2, 9% for B6, and 35% for folic acid
VITAMIN C: 42%
CALCIUM: 60%
COPPER: 13%
VITAMIN E: 13%
FIBER: 6.3 grams
IRON: 22%
MAGNESIUM: 15%
PHOSPHORUS: 9%
POTASSIUM: 490 mg
PROTEIN: 8%

GOOD POINTS

Spinach is low in calories and filled with nutrients. It's an excellent source of vitamin A (as carotene) and vitamin C (both of which can protect you against cancer), folic acid, fiber, and potassium. It also contains magnesium, copper, vitamin E, protein, phosphorus, and other B vitamins. Although spinach has a good amount of iron, only 5% of it is absorbed by the body. It is also high in calcium, but again, only 10% is absorbed

BAD POINTS

Spinach contains significant amounts of sodium. It is also high in NITRATES, which are converted in the body into NITRITES and NITROSAMINES—potential carcinogens (cancer-causing agents). If the spinach is fresh, this is not a problem, but if it is cooked and left standing for some time at room temperature, bacteria that convert nitrates to nitrites multiply and the level of nitrites rises significantly.

It contains GOITROGENS—substances that hamper the production of thyroid hormones by the thyroid gland. This can cause an enlargement of the gland (goiter) in an attempt by the body to compensate for the reduced hormone production by increasing the amount of tissue available. However, people with healthy thyroids would have to eat a very large amount of this vegetable before they would have any kind of problem. This is only of concern for those with sluggish thyroid glands. Goitrogens break down when the vegetable is heated, and so even if you have a thyroid problem, you can eat as much of the cooked vegetable as you want.

SQUASH

Serving Size: ¹/₂ cup (boiled)
Rating:★(summer);★★(winter)

	Winter	Summer
CALORIES:	47.5	14
FAT:	0.1 grams	0.3 grams
SIMPLE CARBOHYDRATE:	11.2 grams	3.1 grams
VITAMIN A:	88%	8%
VITAMIN B2:	7%	5%
VITAMIN C:	17%	17%
FIBER:	1.75 grams	0.6 grams
POTASSIUM:	323 mg	141 mg

GOOD POINTS
Winter squash is an excellent source of vitamin A (as carotene); summer squash also contains some of this immune system-boosting nutrient. Both seasons of the vegetable contain a good amount of vitamin C, as well as potassium. Winter squash is a good source of fiber; the summer variety only contains a little. Both have some vitamin B2. While both are low in calories, summer squash is significantly lower.

BAD POINTS
They both contain a little simple sugar, which can be bad for your teeth.

Squid (Calamari)

Serving Size: 3.5 ounces
Rating:★

CALORIES: 84
CHOLESTEROL: 250 mg
FAT: 1.2 grams
VITAMIN B2: 7%
PHOSPHORUS: 12%
PROTEIN: 36%

GOOD POINTS
Squid is an excellent low-calorie source of protein, a good source of phosphorus, and contains some vitamin B2. However, for health and heart-watchers, it contains one major drawback (see below).

BAD POINTS
It's very high in cholesterol! However, it does contain good amounts of the omega-3 fatty acids, believed to lower cholesterol levels; this can offset some of the harm. Squid can cause ALLERGIC REACTIONS in susceptible people.

Strawberries

Serving Size: 1 cup
Rating:★★

CALORIES: 4
FAT: 0.6 grams
SIMPLE CARBOHYDRATE: 10.5 grams
B COMPLEX VITAMINS: 6% for B2, 5% for B6, 5% for panthothenic acid
VITAMIN C: 142%
FIBER: .8 grams; most of it is in the form of pectin, which can lower blood cholesterol
POTASSIUM: 247 mg

GOOD POINTS
Strawberries are an excellent low-calorie source of vitamin C (needed for healthy gums, teeth, bones,

and muscles), and a good source of potassium (needed for proper muscle contractions, for maintaining the correct fluid balance in the body, to help the transmission of nerve impulses, and for the release of energy from the carbohydrate and protein you eat). They also contain some fiber and B vitamins.

BAD POINTS
Strawberries are often implicated in ALLERGIES. They contain significant amounts of simple carbohydrate, which can contribute to tooth decay.

STURGEON

Serving Size: 3.5 ounces (steamed)
Rating:★★

CALORIES: 160
FAT: 5.7 grams
SODIUM: 108 mg
IODINE: 10%
IRON: 11%
MAGNESIUM: 10%
PHOSPHORUS: 26%
POTASSIUM: 235 mg
PROTEIN: 56%

GOOD POINTS
This fish is an excellent source of protein, required for the growth and maintenance of all your body tissues. It also contains good amounts of phosphorus, potassium, iron, iodine, and magnesium, and is moderately low in calories.

BAD POINTS
Sturgeon contains a little sodium and a little fat.

SUGAR

Serving Size: 1 teaspoon (granular)
Rating: Nope, no stars

CALORIES: 16
FAT: none
SIMPLE CARBOHYDRATE: 4 grams

GOOD POINTS
None, except that it contains no fat.

BAD POINTS
Sugar contains nothing but calories (energy) and can be harmful to your teeth. Brown sugar has traces of other nutrients, but nothing of significance to the body.

SUNFLOWER SEEDS

Serving Size: 1 ounce
Rating:★★

CALORIES: 157
FAT: 13.2 grams
B COMPLEX VITAMINS: 37% for B1, 8% for B3
VITAMIN C: 23%
COMPLEX CARBOHYDRATE: 5.6 grams
VITAMIN E: 48%
FIBER: 1.1 grams
IRON: 11%
PHOSPHORUS: 23%
POTASSIUM: 258 mg
PROTEIN: 10%

GOOD POINTS
These popular snacking seeds are an excellent source of vitamin E and B1, and also contain vitamin C, phosphorus, potassium, protein, iron, fiber, and vitamin B3.

BAD POINTS
Unfortunately, they're also high in calories and fat, although the latter is entirely polyunsaturated and

monounsaturated. While these types tend to lower your blood cholesterol levels, eating any kind of fat seems to raise your risk of contracting breast, uterine, endometrial, ovarian, prostate, and colon cancer.

SWORDFISH

Serving Size: 3.5 ounces (broiled)
Rating:★★★

CALORIES: 156
FAT: 4.0 grams
VITAMIN A: 41%
VITAMIN B3: 55%
IRON: 7%
PHOSPHORUS: 28%
PROTEIN: 62%

GOOD POINTS
Swordfish is an excellent low-fat, low-calorie source of protein, vitamin B3 and vitamin A, all important for the strength of your body's tissues and immune system. It is a very good source of phosphorus and contains some iron. Health-conscious eaters should try to get fish like this into their diets at least three times a week.

BAD POINTS
It contains a small amount of mostly polyunsaturated and monounsaturated fat. Fish is often implicated in ALLERGIC REACTIONS.

SYRUP

Serving Size: 1 tablespoon
Rating: No stars

	CALORIES	FAT	SIMPLE CARBOHYDRATE	POTASSIUM
Cane:	53	none	13.6 grams	85 mg
Corn:	60	none	15 grams	
Maple:	50	none	12.8 grams	

GOOD POINTS
Well, cane syrup does contain a little potassium.

BAD POINTS
Syrup of any kind is mainly empty calories, which come in the form of simple sugars (a contributing factor to tooth decay).

TANGERINE
Serving Size: 1 medium
Rating:★★

CALORIES: 37

FAT: 0.2 grams

SIMPLE CARBOHYDRATE: 9.4

VITAMIN A: 15%

VITAMIN B1: 6%

VITAMIN C: 43%

FIBER: 1.5 grams; most of it is in the form of pectin, which can lower blood cholesterol levels

POTASSIUM: 132 mg

GOOD POINTS
Tangerines are an excellent, low-calorie source of vitamin C, needed for healthy gums, teeth, bones, and muscles. They also contain vitamin A (as carotene), potassium, fiber, and some B1.

BAD POINTS
Tangerines contain a significant amount of simple sugars, which can contribute to tooth decay. Some people develop a rash called CONTACT DERMATITIS from the oils in the skin of the fruit.

TARTAR SAUCE

Serving Size: 1 tablespoon
Rating: Sorry, no stars

CALORIES: 70
CHOLESTEROL: 5 mg
FAT: 7.9 grams
SODIUM: 185 mg

GOOD POINTS
None.

BAD POINTS:
It is high in fat, and although this is mainly of the polyunsaturated and monounsaturated type and so tends to lower blood cholesterol levels, eating any sort of fat appears to raise your risk of getting breast, uterine, endometrial, ovarian, prostate, and colon cancer. It is also high in calories, and contains some cholesterol. This is not a great food choice at all; there are only drawbacks and no benefits in adding gobs of tartar sauce to you fish.

TEA

Serving Size: 1 cup
Rating:★

FAT: none
FLUORIDE: 0.3 - 0.5 mg
FOLIC ACID: 5% (for green tea)
POTASSIUM: 58 mg

GOOD POINTS
Tea contains some folic acid, potassium, and fluoride (which protects your teeth). Green tea has the most folic acid, black teas a little less, and oolong teas have about one-third the amount of green tea.

BAD POINTS
Teas contain up to 50 mg of CAFFEINE per cup; the longer the tea brews the higher the caffeine content.

Substances in tea called TANNINS bind to calcium and iron, preventing the body from absorbing them. Tannins also reduce vitamins B1 and B12 absorption, and may be constipating.

TOFU

Serving Size: 3.5 ounces
Rating:★★

CALORIES: 72
FAT: 4.2 grams
CALCIUM: 13%
IRON: 10%
MAGNESIUM:28%
PHOSPHORUS: 13%
PROTEIN: 17%

GOOD POINTS
Tofu (soy bean curd) is a very good source of magnesium, essential for bone growth, the manufacture of body proteins, the liberation of energy from carbohydrates, and the workings of the nerves and muscles. It is also low in calories, a good source of protein, calcium, and phosphorus, and contains some iron.

BAD POINTS
Tofu contains some fat. Since it is in the form of monounsaturated and polyunsaturated fat it tends to lower your blood cholesterol levels, but any fat seems to raise your risk of breast, uterine, endometrial, ovarian, prostate, and colon cancer. Some people are ALLERGIC to soy protein.

TOMATO

Serving Size: 1 small
Rating:★★★

CALORIES: 14
FAT: 0.2 grams
VITAMIN A: 18%
B COMPLEX VITAMINS: 6% for B6, 7% for folic acid
VITAMIN C: 38%
COPPER: 5%
VITAMIN E: 8%
FIBER: 1.5 grams
POTASSIUM: 290 mg

GOOD POINTS

Tomatoes are an excellent low-calorie source of vitamin C, needed for healthy gums, teeth, bones, and muscles. They are a good source of vitamin A (as carotene), potassium, and fiber, and also contain some copper, vitamin E, vitamins B6, and folic acid. No salad dish is complete without some ripe red tomatoes on top!

BAD POINTS
None.

TROUT

Serving Size: 3.5 ounces (steamed)
Rating:★★

CALORIES: 135
CHOLESTEROL: 80 mg
FAT: 4.5 grams
SODIUM: 88 mg
VITAMIN B3: 6%
IRON: 6%
MAGNESIUM: 8%
PHOSPHORUS: 27%
POTASSIUM: 370 mg
PROTEIN: 52%

GOOD POINTS

Trout is an excellent low-calorie source of protein, required for the growth and maintenance of all body tissues. It also contains phosphorus, potassium, iron, vitamin B3, and magnesium.

BAD POINTS

It's high in cholesterol and contains some fat. Since the fat is mainly monounsaturated and polyunsaturated it tends to lower your blood cholesterol levels, but any fat seems to raise your risk of getting breast, uterine, endometrial, ovarian, prostate, and colon cancer. On the other hand, trout also contains a good amount of the omega-3 fatty acids, also believed to lower blood cholesterol. It contains some sodium. Fish is a common cause of ALLERGIC REACTIONS.

TUNA, CANNED

Serving Size: 3.25 ounces (white in water or oil)

Rating:★★★(water); ★★(oil)

	Water	Oil
CALORIES:	118	190
CHOLESTEROL:	32 mg	21 mg
FAT:	1.75 grams	10 grams
SODIUM:	371 mg	385 mg
VITAMIN B3:	57%	56%
VITAMIN B6:	17%	56%
VITAMIN B12:	22%	29%
IRON:	6%	4%
MAGNESIUM:	8%	8%
PHOSPHORUS:	20%	25%
POTASSIUM:	239 mg	253 mg
PROTEIN:	57%	56%

GOOD POINTS

Tuna is an excellent low-calorie source of protein and vitamin B3. It contains significant amounts of vitamin B12, phosphorus, potassium, B6, magnesium, and iron. Of course, it is much healthier if packed in water than oil.

BAD POINTS
If canned in oil, it is high in fat. Since the fat is mainly monounsaturated and polyunsaturated it tends to lower your blood cholesterol levels, but any fat seems to raise your risk of breast, uterine, endometrial, ovarian, prostate, and colon cancer. Both types (canned in water and oil) contain some cholesterol and are high in sodium. Fish can cause ALLERGIC REACTIONS in susceptible people.

TUNA, FRESH

Serving Size: 3 ounces (cooked)
Rating: ★★★

CALORIES: 157
CHOLESTEROL: 42 mg
SODIUM: 43 mg
FAT: 5.3 mg
VITAMIN B3: 45%
VITAMIN B6: 23%
VITAMIN B12: 154%
IRON: 6%
MAGNESIUM: 8%
PHOSPHORUS: 27%
POTASSIUM: 275 mg
PROTEIN: 56%

GOOD POINTS
Fresh tuna is an excellent low calorie source of protein, vitamin B3 and vitamin B12. It contains significant amounts of vitamin B6, phosphorus, potassium, magnesium, and iron.

BAD POINTS
Fresh tuna contains moderate amounts of sodium, cholesterol and some fat. Since the fat is mainly monounsaturated and polyunsaturated it tends to lower your blood cholesterol levels, but any fat seems to raise your risk of breast, uterine, endometrial,

ovarian, prostate, and colon cancer. Fish can cause ALLERGIC REACTIONS in susceptible people.

TURKEY

Serving Size: 3.5 ounces (roasted)
Rating: ★★★ (without skin)
★★(with skin)

	White Meat (w/o skin)	Dark Meat (w/o skin)
CALORIES:	157	187
FAT:	3.2 grams	7.2 grams
CHOLESTEROL:	69 mg	85 mg
SODIUM:	64 mg	79 mg
VITAMIN B2:	8%	14%
VITAMIN B3:	34%	18%
VITAMIN B6:	28%	18%
VITAMIN B12:	6%	6%
PANTOTHENIC ACID:	7%	13%
COPPER:	2%	8%
IRON:	8%	13%
MAGNESIUM:	7%	6%
PHOSPHORUS:	22%	20%
POTASSIUM:	305 mg	290 mg
PROTEIN:	66%	64%
ZINC:	14%	8%

GOOD POINTS
Turkey is an excellent source of protein and a very good source of B complex vitamins, phosphorus, and potassium. It also contains zinc, iron, magnesium, and copper. White meat is a better source of B3 and B6 than dark meat, but dark meat has more B2, zinc, iron, and pantothenic acid. Dark meat is higher in calories because of its higher fat content, but neither type is a hazard for dieters.

BAD POINTS
Turkey is quite high in fat and cholesterol, with dark meat containing more fat than white meat. If you eat the skin you increase your fat intake by about 5 grams per serving. The fat in turkey is higher in

unsaturated fatty acids than beef but has the same amount of cholesterol. Eating any type of fat appears to increase your cancer risk. Turkey also contains a little sodium.

TURNIP

Serving Size: ²/₃ cup (cooked)
Rating: ★★

CALORIES: 16
FAT: 0.2 grams
VITAMIN C: 37%
FIBER: .9 grams; most of it is in the form of pectin, which can lower blood cholesterol levels
POTASSIUM: 188 mg

GOOD POINTS
Turnips are very low in calories, an excellent source of vitamin C (needed for healthy gums, teeth, bones, and muscles), and a good source of potassium (needed for proper muscle contractions, for maintaining the correct fluid balance in the body, to help the transmission of nerve impulses, and for the release of energy from the carbohydrate and protein you eat). They also contain a little fiber.

BAD POINTS
Turnips contain GOITROGENS—substances that hamper the production of thyroid hormones by the thyroid gland. This can cause an enlargement of the gland (goiter) in an attempt by the body to compensate for the reduced hormone production by increasing the amount of tissue available. However, people with healthy thyroids would have to eat a very large amount of these vegetables before they would have any kind of problem. This is only of concern for those with sluggish thyroid glands. Goitrogens break down when the vegetable is heated, and so even if you have a thyroid problem, you can eat as much of the cooked vegetable as you want.

VEAL

Serving Size: 3.5 ounces (cooked)
Rating: ★★

CALORIES: 277
CHOLESTEROL: 90 mg
FAT: 15.0 grams
SODIUM: 54 mg
B COMPLEX VITAMINS: 8% for B1, 19% for B2, 32%
    for B3, 16% for B6, and 17% for B12
IRON: 23%
MAGNESIUM: 6%
PHOSPHORUS: 29%
POTASSIUM: 527 mg
PROTEIN: 74%

GOOD POINTS
Veal is an excellent source of protein, potassium, and vitamin B3. It also contains B12, phosphorus, iron, B6, B1, and magnesium.

BAD POINTS
Veal is high in saturated fat, cholesterol, and calories, but lower in fat (and higher in protein) than beef from older animals. (Veal is meat from cattle under three months of age and under 400 pounds in weight.) It also contains some sodium.

WALNUTS

Serving Size: 12 halves
Rating: ★

CALORIES: 79
FAT: 7.7 grams
FIBER: .75 mg
MAGNESIUM: 5%
PHOSPHORUS: 8%
POTASSIUM: 104 mg

GOOD POINTS
Walnuts contain significant amounts of potassium, magnesium, phosphorus, and fiber.

BAD POINTS

These nuts are high in calories and fat. Since the fat is almost all monounsaturated and polyunsaturated it tends to lower your blood cholesterol levels, but eating any type of fat seems to raise your risk of breast, uterine, endometrial, ovarian, prostate, and colon cancer. Nuts are often implicated in ALLERGIC REACTIONS.

WATERCRESS

Serving Size: 10 sprigs
Rating: ★

CALORIES: 14%
FAT: none
VITAMIN A: 10%
VITAMIN C: 13%

GOOD POINTS

This garnish or salad green is a good source of vitamin A (needed for healthy skin, hair, and eyes, and to help protect the body from respiratory and gastrointestinal tract cancer), and vitamin C (needed for healthy gums, teeth, bones, and muscles).

BAD POINTS

Watercress contains some NITRATES, which are converted in the body into NITRATES and NITROSAMINES—potential carcinogens (cancer-causing agents).

WHEAT GERM

Serving Size: 1 ounce (¹/₄ cup)
Rating: ★★★

CALORIES: 108
FAT: 3 grams
B COMPLEX VITAMINS: 31% for B1, 14% for B2, 8% for B3, 14% for B6 and 25% for folic acid.

COPPER: 9%
COMPLEX CARBOHYDRATE: 14.1 grams
VITAMIN E: 36%
FIBER: 0.7 grams
IRON: 14%
MAGNESIUM: 23%
PHOSPHORUS: 33%
POTASSIUM: 268 mg
PROTEIN: 13%
ZINC: 32%

GOOD POINTS
Wheat germ is an excellent source of many nutrients—some B vitamins, vitamin E, phosphorus and zinc—and a very good source of magnesium, potassium, and folic acid. It also contains good amounts of protein, iron, fiber, and copper. It is neither very high nor low in calories.

BAD POINTS
It contains some fat. Since it is monounsaturated and polyunsaturated it tends to lower your blood cholesterol levels, but eating any type of fat seems to raise your risk of breast, uterine, endometrial, ovarian, prostate, and colon cancer.

It also contains a substance called GLUTEN which can cause an upset digestive system, anemia, weight loss, bone pain, skin problems, and water retention in people with a condition known as celiac disease.

WHITEFISH
Serving Size: 3.5 ounces (raw)
Rating: ★★

CALORIES: 155
FAT: 8.2 grams
SODIUM: 52 mg
VITAMIN A: 45%
B COMPLEX VITAMINS: 9% for B1, 7% for B2,l 15% for B3
PHOSPHORUS: 27%

POTASSIUM: 299 mg
PROTEIN: 42%

GOOD POINTS

This appetizing fish is an excellent source of vitamin A, needed for healthy skin, hair, and eyes, and to help protect the body from respiratory and gastrointestinal tract cancer, and protein, required for the growth and maintenance of all your body tissues. It also contains good amounts of phosphorus, potassium, and several B complex vitamins. It is neither very high nor low in calories.

BAD POINTS

It is very high in fat (although it contains a good amount of the omega-3 fatty acids, believed to lower blood cholesterol levels). Since it is in the form of monounsaturated and polyunsaturated fat it tends to lower your blood cholesterol levels, but any fat seems to raise your risk of breast, uterine, endometrial, ovarian, prostate, and colon cancer.

Whitefish also contains some sodium. If it is smoked, this process adds CARCINOGENS (cancer-causing agents) along with increasing the sodium content. ALLERGIES to fish are not uncommon.

WINE

Serving Size: 1 glass
Rating: Sorry, no stars

CALORIES: 80 (white); 76 (red)
FAT: none
IRON: 3% mg (white); 15 mg (red)
POTASSIUM: 84 mg (white); 116 mg (red)

GOOD POINTS

Wine contains some potassium and iron.

BAD POINTS

A glass of wine is relatively high in calories. In addition to containing few nutrients, the alcohol content DEPLETES THE BODY of vitamins A, B1,

B2, B6, D, folic acid, calcium, magnesium, zinc, and glucose. Red wines (especially chianti) contain significant amounts of a substance called TYRAMINE, which can be very dangerous when consumed by someone who is taking monoamine oxidase inhibitors (MAOI's), a group of antidepressant medications.

YOGURT
(LOW FAT)

Serving Size: 1 cup
Rating: ★★★

	Plain	Fruit-Flavored
CALORIES:	144	225
CHOLESTEROL:	14 mg	10 mg
FAT:	3.5 grams	2.6 grams
SIMPLE CARBOHYDRATE:	16 grams	42.3 grams
SODIUM:	159 mg	121 mg
VITAMIN B1:	7%	5%
VITAMIN B2:	29%	22%
VITAMIN B6:	6%	4%
VITAMIN B12:	21	16%
FOLIC ACID:	6%	5%
PANTOTHENIC ACID:	13%	10%
CALCIUM:	42%	31%
IODINE:	69%	69%
MAGNESIUM:	10%	8%
PHOSPHORUS:	33%	25%
POTASSIUM:	531 mg	402 mg
ZINC:	13%	10%

GOOD POINTS
Yogurt is an excellent source of potassium, iodine, calcium, and phosphorus, and contains good amounts of protein, B vitamins, magnesium, and zinc. Plain yogurt has the highest amount of these nutrients and the lowest calories; fruit yogurt has the fewest nutrients and the most calories; and coffee, lemon, or vanilla-flavored are between the two ex-

tremes. Yogurt on the whole is not very high in calories, but not as low as some people think, either.

BAD POINTS
Yogurt contains some fat (mainly saturated) and cholesterol. It also contains a lot of simple sugar (which can be bad for your teeth) and quite a lot of sodium.

Some people don't have an enzyme called lactase in their bodies, which is needed to break down milk sugar (lactose). As a result, when they eat dairy products, the lactose passes through the digestive system where it is broken down by bacteria instead, causing flatulence, bloating, and diarrhea. Allergies to the protein in milk, causing symptoms similar to those of lactose intolerance, also affect many people.

ZUCCHINI
Serving Size: ¹/₂ (frozen)
Rating: ★

CALORIES: 16
FAT: 0.2 grams
VITAMIN A: 9%
VITAMIN C: 7%
FIBER: 0.5 grams; some of it is in the form of pectin, which can lower blood cholesterol levels
POTASSIUM: 207 mg

GOOD POINTS
This is an extremely low-calorie vegetable with significant amounts of vitamin A as carotene, needed for healthy skin, hair, and eyes, and to help protect the body from respiratory and gastrointestinal tract cancer. It is also a good source of vitamin C, potassium, and fiber.

BAD POINTS
None.

Sources

The American Dietetic Association. *Handbook of Clinical Dietetics*. New Haven and London: Yale University Press, 1981.

Morgan, Brian L.G. *Nutrition Prescription*. New York: Crown Publishers, Inc., 1987.

Paul, A.A., and Southgate, D.A.T. *McCance and Widdowson's The Composition of Foods*, 4th ed. London: Her Majesty's Stationery Office, 1978.

Pennington, J.A.T. *Bowes and Church's Food Values of Portions Commonly Used*, rev. 15th ed. Philadelphia: J. B. Lippincott Company, 1989.

Shils, M.E., and Young, V., eds. *Modern Nutrition in Health and Disease*. Philadelphia: Lea & Febiger, 1988.

United States Department of Agriculture, prepared by Adams, C.F., *Handbook of the Nutritional Value of Foods in Common Units*. New York: Dover Publications, Inc., 1986.